VENOUS DISORDERS

A Manual of Diagnosis and Treatment

G. Belcaro

Cardiovascular Institute, Chieti University, Italy; and
Academic Vascular Surgery and Irvine Laboratory, St Mary's Hospital, London, UK

A. N. Nicolaides

Academic Vascular Surgery and Irvine Laboratory, St Mary's Hospital, London, UK

M. Veller

University of Witwatersrand, Johannesburg, South Africa

W.B. Saunders Company Ltd

London Philadelphia Toronto Sydney Tokyo

*This book is dedicated to John T. Hobbs
and to Eugene F. Bernstein*

W.B. Saunders
Company Ltd

24–28 Oval Road
London NW1 7DX, UK

The Curtis Center
Independence Square West
Philadelphia, PA 19106–3399, USA

Harcourt Brace & Company
55 Horner Avenue
Toronto, Ontario M8Z 4X6, Canada

Harcourt Brace & Company, Australia
30–52 Smidmore Street
Marrickville, NSW 2204, Australia

Harcourt Brace & Company, Japan
Ichibancho Central Building
22–1 Ichibancho
Chiyoda-ku, Tokyo 102, Japan

© 1995 W.B. Saunders Company Ltd

This book is printed on acid-free paper

A catalogue record for this book is available from the British Library

ISBN 0–7020–2016–8

Typesetting and page make up by Eric Drewery
Printed and bound in Great Britain by the University Press, Cambridge

Contents

List of contributors

G. Belcaro, Cardiovascular Institute, Chieti University, Italy; and Irvine Laboratory, Academic Vascular Surgery, St Mary's Hospital Medical School, London, UK

M. R. Cesarone, Cardiovascular Institute, Chieti University, Italy

M. T. De Sanctis, Cardiovascular Institute, Chieti University, Italy

B. Eklof, Straub Pacific Health Foundation, Honolulu, Hawaii, USA

C. Fisher, Department of Surgery, Royal North Shore Hospital, St Leonards, New South Wales, Australia

G. Goren, Vein Disorder Center, Encino, California, USA

L. Incandela, Cardiovascular Institute, Chieti University, Italy

M. Labropoulos, Irvine Laboratory, Academic Vascular Surgery, St Mary's Hospital Medical School, London, UK

G. Laurora, Cardiovascular Institute, Chieti University, Italy

M. Leon, Irvine Laboratory, Academic Vascular Surgery, St Mary's Hospital Medical School, London, UK

A. N. Nicolaides, Irvine Laboratory, Academic Vascular Surgery, St Mary's Hospital Medical School, London, UK

G. Ramaswami, Irvine Laboratory, Academic Vascular Surgery, St Mary's Hospital Medical School, London, UK

O. Thulesius, Institute of Clinical Physiology, Faculty of Health Sciences, University Hospital, Linköping, Sweden

J. Vale, Department of Urology, St Mary's Hospital, London, UK

S. Vasdekis, Department of Surgery, University of Athens, Greece

M. Veller, Department of Surgery, University of Witwatersrand, Parktown, Johannesburg, South Africa

R. Venniker, Department of Surgery, St Augustine's Hospital, Durban, South Africa

Foreword

The Vascular Laboratory at St Mary's Hospital was founded by Professor Bill Irvine when I returned from Boston, USA in 1961. The initial interest was peripheral arterial disease. In 1963 we took part in the Department of Health trials investigating the treatment of varicose veins. This resulted in the random trial, comparing surgery and sclerotherapy and began an on-going interest in venous disease, encompassing all methods of investigation and expanding the therapeutic options.

The laboratory rapidly grew after the arrival of Andrew Nicolaides who was soon appointed Director and enthusiastically extended our worldwide connections. To accommodate the widening fields of research "metastases" began to appear throughout the hospital. A succession of notable research fellows have passed through the laboratory acquiring higher degrees and extending the work in all areas of vascular physiology and pathology.

The first Doppler instrument (Parks 801) was introduced in 1968 when Jimmy Yao established the ankle/brachial pressure ratio. The directional Doppler soon followed and this instrument was also used to study venous disease. Later duplex instruments with colour imaging appeared and we now eagerly await the imminent arrival of a three-dimension duplex.

The many research fellows have returned to all parts of the globe to continue their interest in vascular diseases. Gianni Belcaro returned to his native Italy in 1984 but since then has returned for one week each month to continue his work in London.

This book is the product of these endeavours and is based on a long time study of venous physiology and pathology. It will provide a good foundation for anyone becoming interested in venous disease. It will be useful for undergraduate students and especially for postgraduate students, surgeons in training and vascular technologists. It will also provide a valuable reference source for physicians dealing with venous problems and dermatologists who have to manage the complications of chronic venous disease.

John T Hobbs
London, 1995

About the Authors

Gianni V. Belcaro graduated in medicine and surgery in 1976. He did his postgraduate research in vascular surgery and physiology at the Bispebjerg Hospital in Copenhagen and in other European centres, including St Mary's Hospital in London where he spent a year as a British Council Scholar. He completed his postgraduate training in general surgery in 1982 and in thoracic surgery in 1989. Since 1983 he has worked at the Cardiovascular Institute of Chieti and in London where he continues to be involved in research at the Irvine Laboratory at St Mary's Hospital.

Martin Veller did his undergraduate training at the University of Witwatersrand, graduating in 1979 and continuing his postgraduate training in general surgery, graduating MMed (Surg) in 1989. He was admitted as a Fellow of the College of Surgeons of South Africa in 1988. He worked for a year in the Irvine Laboratory for Cardiovascular Investigation at St Mary's Hospital in London and since 1992 has been head of the Vascular Surgery Unit in the Department of Surgery at the University of Witwatersrand.

Andrew Nicolaides is Professor of Vascular Surgery at St Mary's Hospital Medical School and enjoys an international reputation because of his work in non-invasive investigations into chronic venous insufficiency. In 1976 he was awarded the Jacksonian Prize of the Royal College of Surgeons for his work on the prevention of postoperative venous thromboembolism. He is President of the International Union of Angiology and Organiser of the Consensus Meetings on Venous Thromboembolism (Windsor, 1991 and London, 1994).

Acknowledgements

Many thanks to all my friends working at the Irvine Laboratory, St Mary's Hospital, particularly to Surinder Dhanjil, Maura Griffin and Jenny Sano. I have also had great help and support from all my collaborators in Pescara, particularly Beatrice and Barbara. Special thanks to Prof. A. Barsotti, Director of the Cardiovascular Institute, Chieti University, for his suggestions and continuous support.

Gianni Belcaro

Published with a contribution from the MURST (Italian Ministry for Scientific and Technological Research).

Anatomy and dynamics of the venous and lymphatic systems

VENOUS ANATOMY

GENERAL CONSIDERATIONS

Venous anatomy has *peripheral* and *central* components, the former containing valves which modulate pressure effects under changing conditions, while the latter are a reservoir which is hydrodynamically continuous. The peripheral component is located principally in the limbs, the integument and organs such as the testes which are outwith the body cavities. The central component includes veins from the intra-abdominal and intrathoracic organs, those that drain the central nervous system as well as the large confluent vessels (iliacs, subclavians, jugulars, brachiocephalic and the inferior and superior vena cavae) that ultimately return blood to the heart. This account is chiefly devoted to the lower limb because of the clinical importance of disorders such as varicose veins but other areas will be considered where they impinge on venous disorders.

LOWER LIMB

The veins of the leg are classified anatomically into two groups: superficial and deep. The two are connected by perforating (communicating) veins that pass through the deep fascia and also at the terminations of the two subdivisions of the superficial system—the saphenofemoral and saphenopopliteal junctions. Within the deep system are muscular veins which, below the knee, drain the gastrocnemius and soleus muscles of the calf and are sinusoidal in character.

Superficial veins

The superficial veins are the long and short saphenous systems (**Figures 1.1, 1.2** and **1.3**). The term *saphenous* is probably a derivative of the Greek word *saphis*—'clearness'—perhaps because the superficial course of the veins make them very evident.

The long saphenous vein (LSV), the longest in the body, begins in front of the medial malleolus, ascends through the medial part of the leg and thigh and terminates by entering the common femoral vein through the saphenous opening in the deep fascia of the groin. The LSV receives several tributaries of which the most important are:

Below the knee

◆ The posterior arch vein (Leonardo's) which joins the LSV at the

Figure 1.1 The long saphenous system and the deep venous system. For detailed consideration see text.

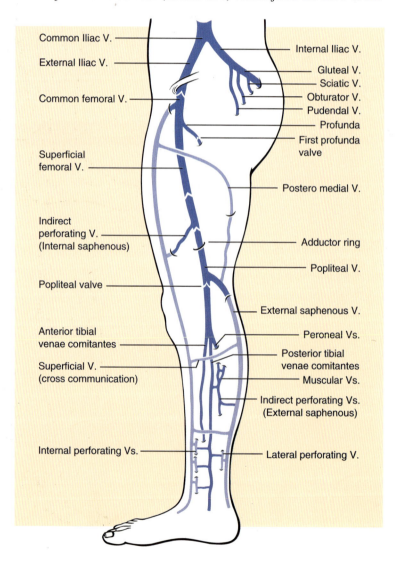

Common Iliac V.

External Iliac V.

Common femoral V.

Superficial femoral V.

Indirect perforating V. (Internal saphenous)

Popliteal valve

Anterior tibial venae comitantes

Superficial V. (cross communication)

Internal perforating Vs.

Internal Iliac V.

Gluteal V.

Sciatic V.

Obturator V.

Pudendal V.

Profunda

First profunda valve

Postero medial V.

Adductor ring

Popliteal V.

External saphenous V.

Peroneal Vs.

Posterior tibial venae comitantes

Muscular Vs.

Indirect perforating Vs. (External saphenous)

Lateral perforating V.

medial aspect of the knee. Its importance lies in its connection to the deep venous system by two or three relatively constant perforating veins at the posterior margin of the medial border of the tibia between the malleolus and the medial condyle (Cockett's perforators – see **Figure 1.2** and p. 5).

◆ The anterior superficial tibial vein which joins the long saphenous at the same level as the posterior arch vein.

Figure 1.2 The long saphenous system and the internal ankle perforating veins. For detailed consideration see text.

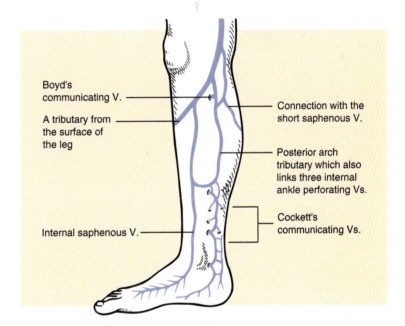

Boyd's communicating V.

A tributary from the surface of the leg

Internal saphenous V.

Connection with the short saphenous V.

Posterior arch tributary which also links three internal ankle perforating Vs.

Cockett's communicating Vs.

Figure 1.3 External saphenous vein and the constant perforating veins.

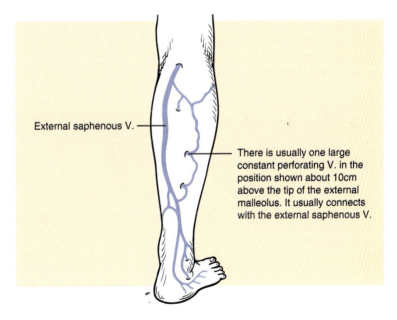

External saphenous V.

There is usually one large constant perforating V. in the position shown about 10cm above the tip of the external malleolus. It usually connects with the external saphenous V.

Above the knee

◆ The anterolateral and posteromedial veins are two long tributaries that are variably present and join the LSV near its termination. The posteromedial vein often connects with the upper part of the short saphenous vein (SSV) just before the latter penetrates the deep fascia.

◆ Tributaries that join the long saphenous at the level of its junction with the deep system are the superficial circumflex iliac, the superficial inferior epigastric and the superficial external pudendal. The anatomy is very varied at this point and is of importance when the saphenofemoral junction is interrupted at surgery.

The short saphenous vein (SSV) begins at the outer border of the foot behind the lateral malleolus and ascends approximately in the posterior midline of the calf to the popliteal fossa where it pierces the deep fascia to join the popliteal vein. The level of termination is variable with more than 30% ending high up in the thigh.

Deep veins The deep veins below the knee are three paired stems which run as
(Figure 1.1) venae comitantes along the corresponding arteries—anterior tibial, posterior tibial and the peroneal (fibular). The posterior tibial veins receive the important medial ankle (Cockett's) perforators from the posterior arch vein. The stem veins merge at the upper part of the calf to form the popliteal vein. This ascends through the opening in the adductor magnus to become the superficial femoral vein in the adductor (subsartorial) canal. Occasionally one head of origin of the gastrocnemius muscle partially encircles the popliteal vein and this may cause *popliteal entrapment* (see p. 170). The deep femoral vein joins the superficial femoral vein approximately 9 cm below the inguinal ligament to form the common femoral. This continues upwards and, as it passes posterior to the inguinal ligament, becomes the external iliac vein.

There are considerable variations in the anatomy of the deep veins. It has been suggested that the classical anatomical pattern is present in only 16% of limbs.

The muscle veins drain the gastrocnemius and soleus muscles. There are usually two gastrocnemius veins, one draining each head of the gastrocnemius muscle though the medial one is frequently double. They terminate by joining the popliteal vein at the same level as does the short saphenous. In about a third of instances the confluence with the popliteal vein is common to all the tributaries. The variations in the anatomy and the communications of the veins with others in the popliteal fossa can be demonstrated by venography. Distally the gastrocnemius veins communicate with the SSV through a midcalf perforating vein at the site often known as the *gastrocnemius point*.

The veins which drain the soleus muscle are large, sausage-shaped vessels devoid of valves and in consequence are sometimes called the *soleal sinusoids*. They join the posterior tibial and peroneal veins or the more distal part of the popliteal vein.

Perforating or communicating veins (Figures 1.1 to 1.3) These pierce the deep fascia to connect the superficial with the deep venous system. The use of the words *perforating* or *communicating* varies from author to author but in the English language literature the two terms are synonymous. Classification is into *direct*—those passing straight from the superficial vein to the main deep veins—or *indirect*—when the connection is via a muscle sinuspid. Extensive anatomical dissections have indicated that more than 100 perforating veins may be present in a limb but very few are of clinical importance.

The main connections of the LSV to the deep veins are from below upwards:

- Cockett's perforating veins are of the greatest clinical importance. They lie on a perpendicular line (Linton's line) behind the medial malleolus and connect the posterior arch veins with the posterior tibial vena comitantes. They are usually three (lower, middle and upper) and are at an average distance of 6, 13.5 and 18.5 cm respectively above the tip of the medial malleolus. In addition to these, another perforating vein may be present above the upper one (the *24 cm perforator*).
- Boyd's perforating vein at the level of the tibial tuberosity connects the main trunk of the LSV with the posterior tibial veins or sometimes with a branch of the gastrocnemius veins.
- Dodd's perforating or thigh perforators are a group of veins which connect the LSV or an accessory LSV with the femoral vein. They can occur at any site on the medial aspect of the thigh but the majority are found in the middle third of the thigh.

Important connections between the SSV and the deep veins include:

- Bassi's perforator, a constant perforating vein which connects the SSV with the peroneal vein approximately 5 cm above the os calcis.
- The soleus point perforator which connects the soleus veins with the superficial veins of the calf.
- The gastrocnemius point perforator or gastrocnemius 'blow-out', to which aching symptoms are ascribed when there is valvular incompetence, connects the gastrocnemius vein with the superficial system (the SSV and its tributaries).

Valves in the lower limb veins

Valves in the veins of the lower extremity are bicuspid, more numerous distally and less common proximally. In addition, the more distal the vein, the thicker is its wall in relation to its potential calibre.

The sites of valves are classified as follows:

◆ between every point of communication between the superficial and deep systems, including the saphenofemoral and saphenopopliteal junctions, so that blood flow is normally from superficial to deep.
◆ in the axial veins of the deep system. There is nearly always a valve in the upper part of the popliteal vein and usually one or more in the superficial femoral vein.
◆ usually in the gastrocnemius veins.

Valves are usually absent from the soleal sinusoids.

UPPER LIMB INCLUDING THE ROOT OF THE NECK (Figure 1.4a–b)

Superficial and deep systems are present in the upper limb in a similar way as to the lower extremity.

Superficial veins

The two main pathways for blood from the skin and subcutaneous systems are the *basilic* and *cephalic*. The former receives blood from the palm and ventral aspect of the forearm and converges on the medial aspect of the elbow where the basilic vein itself penetrates the deep fascia to become the vena comitans of the brachial artery. The latter drains the dorsal surface of hand and arm and passes up the lateral aspect into the bicipital groove where a single channel passes through the costoclavicular membrane to join the axillary vein.

Deep veins

The venae comitantes of the distal axial arteries join to form those of the brachial which receive the basilic vein and usually become a single channel which, as it crosses the posterior fold of the axilla, becomes the axillary vein. The latter has numerous tributaries corresponding to the branches of the axillary artery. This extensive network ensures an alternative route of drainage to the trunk should the axillary vein be blocked.

At the outer border of the first rib the axillary vein becomes the subclavian which crosses above and in front of the rib and behind the clavicle and is then joined by the internal jugular to form the brachiocephalic (innominate) vein. The subclavian vein is separated

Figure 1.4 a,b Veins of the upper limb and root of the neck.

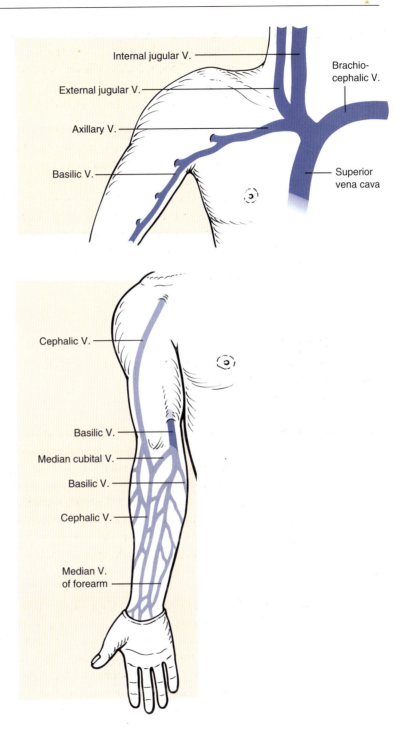

Internal jugular V.

Brachio-cephalic V.

External jugular V.

Axillary V.

Basilic V.

Superior vena cava

Cephalic V.

Basilic V.

Median cubital V.

Basilic V.

Cephalic V.

Median V. of forearm

from the subclavian artery behind by the scalenus anterior muscle which is inserted into the first rib. This narrow pathway is susceptible to compression and may be one predisposing cause of axillary vein thrombosis (see p. 117).

Valves in the veins of the upper arm

As with the lower limb, both the superficial and deep systems in the upper limb contain valves and it was in the former that William Harvey was able to demonstrate the circulation of the blood. The proximal part of the axillary vein contains a pair of valves but these are the last in the upper limb drainage system.

GENITAL ORGANS (Figure 1.5)

In both male and female the initial venous drainage is plexiform. The plexus around the testis is continued proximally as a convoluted collection of veins (the pampiniform plexus) in the spermatic cord. After the cord enters the abdomen this is usually reduced to two veins and then a single channel which runs up the posterior abdominal wall to enter the inferior vena cava on the right and the renal vein on the left. In the female there are intercommunicating plexuses of veins surrounding both the ovary and the uterus. The ovarian drainage is then similar to that of the testis with the veins coalescing into one or two ovarian veins which have a similar anatomical course to the testicular veins. The uterine plexus in the broad ligament becomes two uterine veins which open into the internal iliac veins. Inferiorly, the uterine plexus communicates with the plexus of veins in the vaginal wall and labia which also come together to form vaginal veins which drain into the internal iliacs.

Valves in the genital veins

The spermatic and ovarian vessels contain valves but there are few in the pelvic plexuses or the large veins formed from them.

MICROCIRCULATION

The *venules* that converge to form veins are themselves preceded by the capillary circulation through which tissues are supplied with oxygen and nutrients and relieved of metabolites. Exchange takes place through pores in the capillary membrane. There are two minute passageways serving this function: the intercellular cleft—a thin slit between adjacent endothelial cells; and pinocytic vesicles that carry large molecules.

Figure 1.5 Pelvic venous system and veins of the ovary and testis.

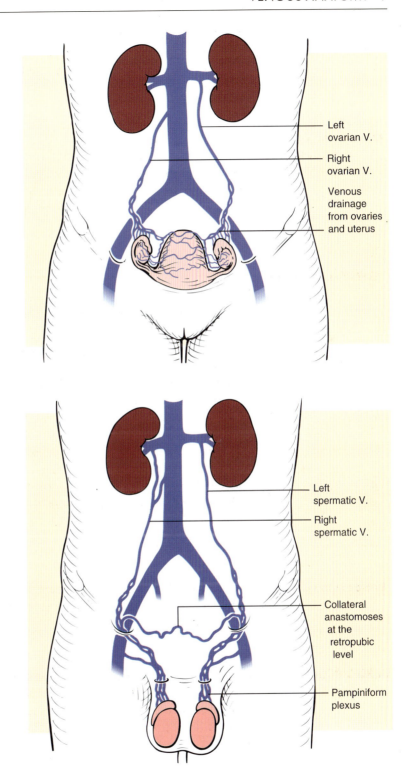

The lymphatic vessels in tissues and the lymph nodes to which they drain are part of a larger system which includes organs such as the spleen concerned with a wide range of functions in the body focused on protection from infection and the recognition of self. However, this account deals mainly with the physical features of the drainage system in that disorders of it are a cause of swollen limbs with which venous disease can be associated or confused.

The most peripheral lymphatic vessels closely resemble the blood capillaries but begin as blind tubes in the tissues, contain valves and form a plexus in the superficial dermis (**Figure 1.6**). They are responsible for the resorption of between 10 and 20% of the interstitial fluid but their much greater permeability to large molecules than that of the blood capillary means that they act as the pathway for transfer of much of the protein and protein debris that accumulates in the interstitial space.

A deep plexus is present in the deeper dermis in the extremities and a subfascial plexus within the muscular compartments. Tissue fluid derived from the capillary system is collected into dermal lymphatics and drains into subcutaneous lymphatics that follow the course of many superficial veins. From there lymphatic flow is into major regional lymphatic channels and clusters of lymph nodes which in the limbs are found in the axilla and inguinal regions. Large lymphatic vessels are usually close to and follow the course of the major blood vessels.

Large lymphatics have some muscle in their wall which indicates contractile power and the numerous delicate endothelial valves they contain direct flow in a central direction only. The lymph nodes, regularly located along the larger lymphatic channels, trap and make available for phagocytosis particles and other matter that has crossed the wall of the lymphatic. Furthermore, they also present foreign material to the immunologically active cells they contain. Two to four litres of lymph (containing between 70 and 200 g of protein) enter the brachiocephalic veins daily through the two final common pathways of the lymphatic system in the root of the neck—the *thoracic duct* on the left and the *right lymphatic duct.*

Muscular contraction during exercise and normal activity, as in the venous system (see p. 14), increases the velocity and therefore the quantity of lymphatic flow. Flow is also raised in the early stages of venous obstruction, in inflammation and infection, in all situations which produce vasodilatation and when there is an

Figure 1.6 Distal lymphatic system. The arteriolar end of the system, the venular end and the capillary loop are shown below. Prelymphatic spaces are indicated by arrows and drain into the lymphatic channels which follow the course of the artery and vein.

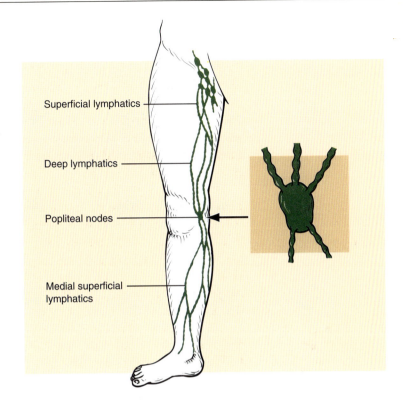

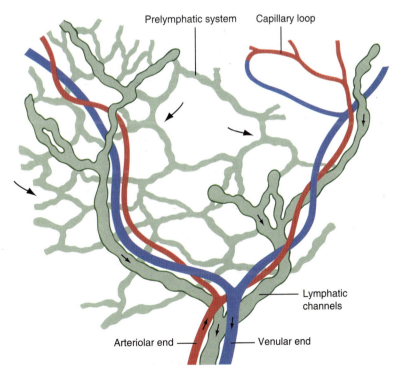

increase in capillary permeability. Obstruction at the clusters of lymph nodes at the roots of the limbs inevitably results in diminished lymphatic drainage because there is little in the way of a collateral lymphatic circulation around these points.

FLUID DYNAMICS OF THE VENOUS SYSTEM

GENERAL The anatomical concept of peripheral and central components of the venous system has already been mentioned and this carries over into a consideration of dynamics. In normal circumstances the pressure within the central part of the venous system is relatively constant: in so far as it varies it does so as a whole, partly under the influence of gravity and partly from changes in intra-abdominal and intrathoracic dynamics, chiefly those produced by breathing. Regions and organs which drain directly into central veins are exposed to this pressure and its variations. By contrast, peripheral regions, such as the limbs and to a lesser extent the genital organs, are protected by valves and thus have different and local hydrodynamics provided their valves remain competent. This is particularly the case in the lower limb which is the main focus of the following account.

LOWER LIMB The venous system of the legs may be dynamically divided into four subsystems which follow the description of the anatomy: superficial, deep, perforating (communicating), and the microcirculation. Malfunction that leads to 'deep venous insufficiency' (for a detailed definition see p. 124) may arise from one or more than one of these subsystems.

The *deep venous system* includes all veins within muscular compartments and beneath the deep fascia. This system returns some 85% of the blood delivered to the leg. The *superficial system* located in the subcutaneous tissue, superficial to the deep fascia, includes the greater and lesser saphenous veins and their tributaries. The *perforating (communicating)* veins connect the two systems by traversing the deep fascia. The valves within them permit flow from superficial to deep veins only.

Venous pressure In normal erect individuals if the mean pressure in the right atrium is taken as zero, hydrostatic pressure in a vein in the superficial venous system such as on the dorsum of the foot would be, when all valves are open, equal to the distance from the right atrium to the foot—about 100–130 cmH$_2$O (73.7–95.8 mmHg). This is indeed largely the case when the individual is at rest with full muscle relaxation. However, at any one moment there is *some* muscle contraction within the semi-rigid compartments deep to the deep fascia which compresses muscular veins, particularly the valveless soleal sinuses, so driving blood proximally towards the heart. This is the important *muscle pump* and is associated with increased flow in the deep veins with intermittent opening and closing of the valves within them. Both of these maintain a relatively low pressure in the deep system which allows blood to move from the superficial to the deep system through competent perforating veins. The more the muscles are relaxed, the less intermittent variation there is in the pressure in the deep venous system and the veins fill passively. By contrast, the more efficient is the muscular action, the lower the level of pressure becomes in the superficial system. This is well illustrated by the changes that occur in superficial venous pressure (SVP) during walking when it falls from a resting value of about 100–120 cmH$_2$O to approximately 30 cmH$_2$O (**Figure 1.7**). The decrease in superficial venous pressure (known as the ambulatory venous pressure, AVP—see also p. 37) is maintained until the end of the exercise, after which the level returns relatively slowly to the pre-exercise value by filling of the venous system from the arterial side.

The dynamics are changed by incompetence of the valves in the communicating veins. At rest, SVP is little different from the relatively high pressure found in the normal limb. However, when, during exercise, there is increased expulsion of blood from the deep sinusoids, a proportion of this *refluxes* from deep to

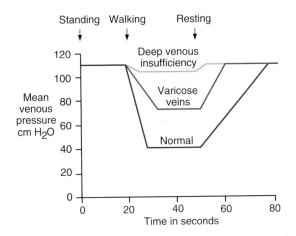

Figure 1.7 Changes in ambulatory venous pressure in a normal subject, a subject with deep venous insufficiency and one with varicose veins. In a normal subject, pressure decreases on walking and gradually rises when this ceases. In patients with incompetence between the deep and superficial systems, pressure decreases much less on walking and returns rapidly to the pre-exercise value.

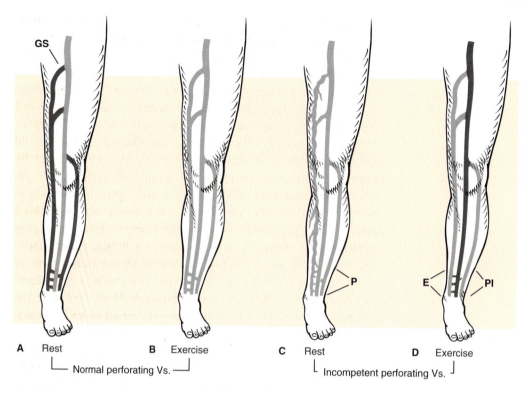

| A | Rest | B | Exercise | C | Rest | D | Exercise |

└— Normal perforating Vs. —┘   └ Incompetent perforating Vs. ┘

Figure 1.8 The normal venous system during standing (A) and walking (B), and dynamic abnormalities in an incompetent system during exercise (C,D). Pressure in the superficial veins is normally decreased during exercise if the valves are competent. The muscular action promotes venous return from the superficial to the deep system, to the proximal veins and towards the heart (B).

C. When the superficial valves are incompetent and the superficial system is varicose (initial superficial incompetence) competence of the distal perforating veins (P) contains venous flow from the superficial to the deep system and venous return during exercise is normal. The efficacy of the calf muscle pump is essentially maintained and the ambulatory venous pressure is only slightly elevated (C).

D. If the valves of the deep system are incompetent in association with incompetence of the valves of the perforating veins (PI) severe chronic venous hypertension develops, leading to oedema, swelling and eventually ulceration.

The problem may be further complicated by the association of deep and superficial incompetence (greater saphenous vein and lesser saphenous vein incompetence).

GS = greater saphenous system; P = normal perforators; PI = perforators incompetence; E = oedema.

Note: Veins with high venous pressure are shown in black.

superficial veins along the incompetent channels though eventually, of course, it must all leave the limb through the main venous channels. In consequence, the SVP does not fall to anything like the same extent and, furthermore, the return to the pre-exercise level when the activity stops (often referred to as the *refilling time*) is more rapid (**Figure 1.8**). Exercise-induced change in SVP and the speed of refilling can thus be used as measures of deep or superficial valvular incompetence. The observation of induced reflux (usually by increasing flow with calf compression) by appropriate imaging provides the same information (see pp. 33–34). Incompetence of valves in the deep system causes somewhat similar effects in that there is now a single column of blood between the right atrium and whatever point in the lower limb is chosen for the measurement of pressure; the muscle pump continues to drive blood proximally but when exercise ceases there is momentary reflux within the deep veins. A combination of valvular incompetence in both systems increases AVP still further during exercise. The quantity of reflux is also increased in such circumstances because there is persistent deep venous hypertension.

Any increased venous pressure is transmitted to the venules so that reabsorption at the venous end of the capillary is impaired. When the increase in pressure has been of long standing, the capillary network is much altered and the changes that take place in it and the overlying skin and subcutaneous tissues are discussed in Chapter 11.

Venous capacitance

As is the case elsewhere in the body, the veins of the lower limb can expand and contract over a wide range as compared with the arteries and so form a capacitance system which contains a variable amount of blood according to the position of the limb, the activity of the muscle pump, the integrity of the venous valves and the overall blood volume. The size and variability of this *venous reservoir* can be studied by the techniques of plethysmography and have come to assume an important role in the assessment of venous disorders (Chapter 4, pp. 40–42).

2 Physiology of veins and their relationship with venous disorders

GENERAL

Veins have three principal functions:

◆ Conduction of blood towards the heart.
◆ Storage of blood.
◆ Thermoregulation.

Conduction

Veins are a very effective, low resistance pathway for the return of blood to the heart. In the extremities there are about three times as many veins as arteries and here, as elsewhere in the body, the drainage network is interconnected. In consequence, a block to or removal of a single vessel usually does not disrupt flow as much as does an arterial occlusion.

Storage

The ability of veins to vary their diameter over a wide range (see p. 18) makes them an important compartment for the storage of blood—their capacitance function. Seventy per cent of the blood volume is in the veins at any one time (**Figure 2.1**). Small changes in venous calibre are important for the regulation of cardiac output by their effect on venous return to and preload of the heart.

Thermoregulation

Dissipation of heat from the core of the body is controlled by diversion of blood flow to the superficial cutaneous veins and heat loss prevented by the opposite process. Heat conservation is also achieved by the *countercurrent heat exchanger* in the deep vessels. Relatively cool venous blood returning from the extremities along the venae comitantes and axial veins adjacent to the arteries gains

Figure 2.1
The relative vascular volumes in the two sections of the circulation.

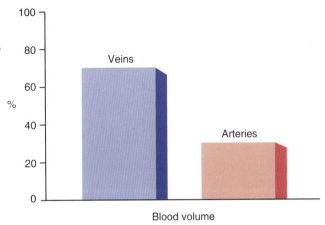

heat from the arterial blood, cooling this in the process. A rise in local and body temperature leads to dilatation of skin veins so that countercurrent exchange is reduced and, by contrast, venoconstriction in response to cold directs blood to the deep veins and so enhances heat transfer.

Thermoregulation is largely controlled by sympathetic venoconstrictor nerves. Normal superficial veins are themselves sensitive to cooling and venoconstriction is also elicited by a very effective mechanism independent of nerve activity but based on the blockade of the sodium-potassium-ATPase sodium pump. This mechanism is inoperative in veins that have become varicose.

ELASTIC PROPERTIES OF VEINS

Direct observation of veins in the subcutaneous tissue gives the impression that they are very distensible—sometimes flaccid and collapsed and at other times distended. However, the normal vein wall is in fact relatively stiff and resists distension which becomes obvious on study of the volume–pressure relationships. During expansion from the collapsed state there is an initial substantial change in volume with little concomitant increase in pressure—characteristic of the *filling phase* which does not involve any stretch of the wall. Once the vein has assumed a circular configuration, further rise in pressure is accompanied by elongation of the components of the wall and the true elastic behaviour of the wall is revealed. The slope of the curve which relates volume and pressure is now an indication of the elastic modulus (**Figure 2.2**) and, if veins and arteries are compared in this way, it becomes evident that the former are not more distensible than arteries.

A further misconception about the elasticity of the vascular wall is the belief that a contracted vessel is less distensible (stiffer) than a relaxed one. Contrary to expectation—based on the association

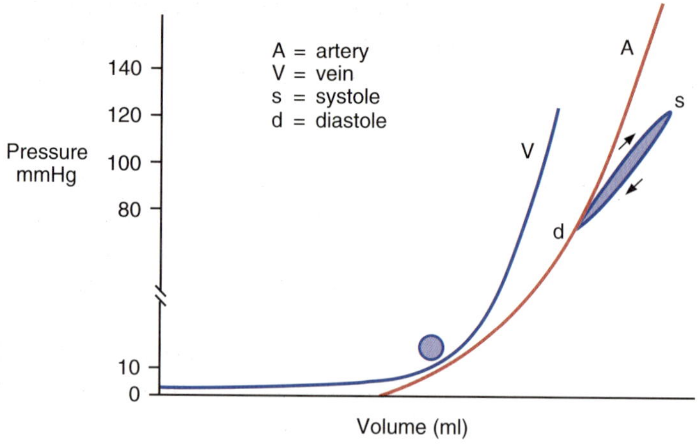

Figure 2.2 Volume–pressure relationship for arterial and venous segments. Note the initial large change in volume of the vein during the filling phase. The steep pressure rise that follows reflects elasticity.

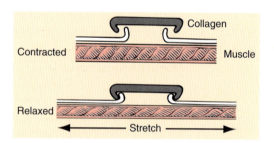

Figure 2.3 Schematic model of the elements of the wall of a vein–collagen and smooth muscle – with and without stretch.

of smooth muscle contraction with increased isometric tension and 'hardening' of the muscle—resistance to deformation is lower in contracted than in relaxed veins because of the inherent flexibility of smooth muscle compared to collagen. In a relaxed and expanded vein, collagen fibres are a supportive 'jacket' that resists further load and it is only in vessels with a large content of elastic fibres, such as medium to large arteries, that distensibility is greater.

To explore this concept further it is necessary to look at the viscoelastic properties of a vein composed of smooth muscle and connective tissue arranged in parallel (**Figure 2.3**). Elongation (length) and stress (tension) are measured as the model is stretched. As already mentioned, the slope of the length–tension curve expresses elasticity (stiffness) of the wall. With the smooth muscle contracted, stretch lengthens the internal elastic elements of the muscle which produces a small value for the slope—the vein is not very stiff. In a dilated vein with the smooth muscle relaxed, the curve is initially of slight slope only because filling is taking place. Thereafter, the wall elements become stretched and the slope increases as the parallel elastic and collagen elements come under stress.

Normal veins exhibit the property of *stress relaxation* or *creep* which is a short-lasting relaxation of the vessel wall in response to abrupt filling. The mechanism is an inherent one of smooth muscle and helps to damp the effect of rapid changes in volume. Stress relaxation is lost in veins that have become varicose.

CONTROL OF VENOUS TONE

As in arteries, veins are supplied by sympathetic – adrenergic vasoconstrictor nerves which induce contraction of smooth muscle. Activation can occur as part of the regulation of blood pressure: venoconstriction increases the return of blood to the heart and, in consequence, cardiac output; venodilatation, by contrast, is associated with an increased quantity of blood in the venous system at a lower pressure so that cardiac output may be reduced with resulting hypotension.

SPECIAL FEATURES OF LARGE VEINS

Larger veins—such as those of the axial system of the lower limb and also the saphenous—have a similar cross-sectional structure as arteries with distinguishable adventitia, media and intima. However, the layers are not as distinctly separated as on the arterial side and elastic fibres are less in evidence. The adventitia is connective tissue and the media contains smooth muscle, the thickness of which varies with the degree of stress to which the wall is exposed. In the lower limb, the amount of smooth muscle increases from proximal to distal so that the wall of a foot vein is thicker than that in the thigh. In consequence, normal veins in the foot and calf develop more active (that is, produced by muscle contraction) tension when stimulated with noradrenaline than do those more proximally (**Figure 2.4**). This is obviously an adaptive process to the upright posture which allows distal veins to withstand higher transmural pressure. Veins in the deep system have a thinner media than those in the superficial system such as the long saphenous but are supported by the fascial boundaries of the muscle compartments.

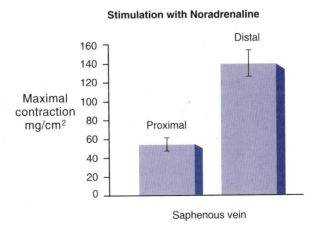

Figure 2.4 Pharmacological properties of normal proximal and distal saphenous vein. There is a higher contractile force and a lower threshold to noradrenaline stimulation in the distal segment in comparison with the proximal segment (proximal threshold 1.1×10^{-6}; distal threshold 2.9×10^{-6} M).

Figure 2.5
Comparison of testing
for competence of the
uppermost valve of the
long saphenous vein in
controls and patients
with varicose veins.
Mean values are
shown. There is a mean
lower leak pressure in
patients but some con-
trols may have a leaky
valve and some patients
a leak pressure within
the normal range.

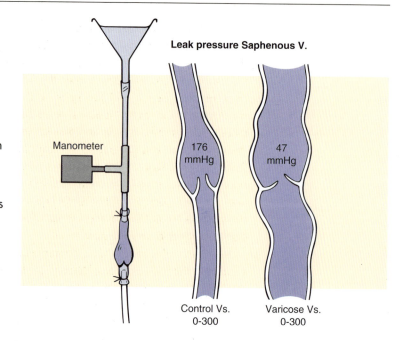

Leak pressure Saphenous V.

Manometer

176 mmHg

47 mmHg

Control Vs.
0-300

Varicose Vs.
0-300

VENOUS VALVES

A key structure in peripheral veins is the venous valve which helps maintain centripetal flow without reflux (see also p. 6). A normal valve is capable of withstanding the hydrostatic pressure imposed on it by the upright position plus the extra load that can be applied in physiological manoeuvres such as abdominal straining against a contracted diaphragm and closed glottis (Valsalva manoeuvre).

Valve integrity can be evaluated by determining the pressure at which leakage occurs with retrograde filling of an isolated vein. Normal veins withstand a remarkably high retrograde pressure in excess of 300 mmHg. When pressure is increased from above the sinus region, the valve characteristically expands so that the vein becomes pear-shaped (**Figure 2.5**). The venous dilatation which takes place during exercise or reactive hyperaemia does not cause reflux in normal veins.

MICROCIRCULATION

Blood flow in the microcirculation is dependent on the arterio-venous pressure difference, the vascular resistance and the viscosity of the blood. Viscosity in turn is a function of the blood cells present and of the composition of the plasma. The higher the ratio of red cells to plasma (the haematocrit) the more viscous is the blood. Changes in the tendency of cells to aggregate and also in their flexibility also influence viscosity. White blood cells (WBCs), though fewer in number, are 2000 times stiffer than are red cells and trapping of WBCs is therefore a possible contributory factor to inadequate circulation through the capillaries.

Postcapillary venules are more numerous than precapillary arterioles and have a large surface area. They play an important part in the exchange of fluid and solutes: when hydrostatic pressure within the capillary-venular loop exceeds the osmotic pressure differential between the plasma and the interstitial space, movement is outwards: once the hydrostatic pressure has fallen to less than the osmotic differential, water and solutes are reabsorbed. The latter is the case at the venular end of the capillary which provides therefore a large absorptive surface for interstitial fluid absorption and thus the prevention of oedema. A rise in venular hydrostatic pressure as may occur in the presence of incompetent valves or obstruction to outflow in the venous circulation disturbs this delicate balance and oedema may result.

Both arterioles and venules contain smooth muscle cells in their walls and the ratio of precapillary to postcapillary resistance is 4:1. An increase in venular tone elevates and precapillary constriction lowers capillary pressure; in addition, the latter reduces capillary surface area. In the erect posture, capillary pressure rises according to the level of hydrostatic pressure produced and fluid filtration therefore increases. Normally these changes are balanced by a venoarterial reflex which increases precapillary tone, so returning capillary pressure, the number of perfused capillaries and the filtration to their original values. In advanced venous disease and diabetic neuropathy this compensatory mechanism is impaired and contributes to fluid accumulation in the interstitium.

Capillary permeability is governed by the integrity of the endothelium and its basal membrane. Endothelial gaps and the interendothelial cell matrix are the main factors which control capillary permeability especially on the venular side. Increased leakage of water, solutes and macromolecules may occur if the capillary wall is damaged. In venous hypertension, trapped and activated polymorphonuclear leucocytes release cytokines such as interleukin-1 and histamine, so initiating an inflammatory reaction which increases permeability.

ENDOTHELIAL FUNCTION

The role of the endothelium in local vasomotor control is clearly established. Endothelial cells in arteries can produced *endothelial derived relaxing factor* (EDRF) which is now known to be nitric oxide (NO). Certain vasoconstrictors—for example noradrenaline and serotonin—stimulate NO production, so modifying their primary effect. Damage to the endothelium therefore enhances the effect of these substances because of the failure to produce NO. However, the situation on the venous side is the opposite: the endothelium in the human saphenous vein facilitates contraction in response to noradrenaline; and removal of the endothelium attenuates vasoconstriction. In varicose veins, the endothelial-mediated enhancement of noradrenaline-induced vasoconstriction is reduced probably because of endothelial damage which has also been documented by functional and ultrastructural studies. Therefore it is possible that local dilatation of veins and the development of varicosities can be initiated by endothelial damage.

LYMPHATIC DRAINAGE

Drainage of interstitial water and solutes and also of macromolecules back into the general circulation is an important function of the lymphatic plexus. Normally, as described on p. 10, this process occurs because of propulsive contraction of the lymphatics, the activity of muscles and the presence of valves. Pressure in the terminal lymphatics in human skin in the supine position varies from -7 to +11 mmHg. In larger lymphatics, intrinsic contractions can produce 'systolic' pressures of 12–70 mmHg (**Figure 2.6**).

Oedema formation is the result of a local accumulation of interstitial fluid but does not become clinically obvious until volume has risen by 20%. The cause varies with the clinical circumstances and may be the outcome of uncompensated venous hypertension, increased capillary permeability or decreased lymphatic drainage.

Figure 2.6 Lymphatic pressure within the skin, the extremities and the thorax. Note zero to negative pressure in the terminal lymphatics of the skin and high pulsatile pressure in the extremities before the barrier of the lymph node is crossed.

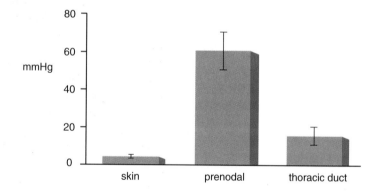

BIBLIOGRAPHY

Aucland K, Reed RK. Interstitial-lymphatic mechanisms in the control of extracellular fluid volume. *Physiol Rev* 1993; **73**: 1–78.

Belcaro G, Nicolaides AN. The predictive value of laser Doppler measurements in diabetic microangiopathy and foot ulcers. In: Bernstein EF. *Vascular Diagnosis*. St Louis: CV Mosby, 1993; 561–7.

Gow BS. The influence of vascular smooth muscle on the visco-elastic properties of blood vessels. In: Bergel DH, ed. *Cardiovascular Fluid Dynamics*. London, 1972; Vol 2, pp. 65–110.

Hendrikson O. Local sympathetic reflex mechanism in regulation of blood flow in subcutaneous adipose tissue. *Acta Physiol Scand* 1977; suppl 450.

Olszewski WL, Engeset A. Intrinsic contractility of prenodal lymph vessels and lymph flow in human leg. *Am J Physiol* 1980; **239**: H755–38.

Spiegel M, Vesti B, Shore A, Franzeck UK, Becker F, Bollinger A. Pressure of lymphatic capillaries in human skin. *Am J Physiol* 1992; **262**: H1208–10

Thulesius O, Gjores JE. Reactions of venous smooth muscle in normal men and patients with varicose veins. *Angiology* 1974; **25**: 145–54.

Thulesius O, Yousif MH. Na^+,K^+-ATPase inhibition, a new mechanism for cold-induced vasoconstriction in cutaneous veins. *Acta Physiol Scand* 1990; **141**: 127–8.

Thulesius O, *et al.* Functional study of isolated venous valves with special comments on the etiology of varicose veins. *American European Symposium on Venous Diseases* 1974; 74-6.

Thulesius O, *et al.* The varicose saphenous vein, functional and ultrastructural studies, with special reference to smooth muscle. *Phlebology* 1988; **3**: 89–95.

Thulesius O, Ugaily-Thulesius L, Neglen P, Shuhaiber H. The role of the endothelium in the control of venous tone: studies on isolated human veins. *Clin Physiol* 1988; **8**: 359–66.

Thulesius O, Said S, Shuhaiber H, Neglen P, Gjores JE. Endothelial mediated enhancement of noradrenalin induced vasoconstriction in normal and varicose veins. *Clin Physiol* 1991; **11**: 153–9.

Diseases of the venous and lymphatic systems – an overview

This chapter gives an overview of the disorders and diseases of the venous and lymphatic systems from the clinical point of view and directs the reader towards the more detailed consideration in other sections of the book.

The swollen limb (Chapter 12) is a frequent observation and often the first sign in venous and lymphatic diseases. Swelling and oedema are associated with either increased production or decreased removal of interstitial fluid or a combination of both. Impaired venous drainage in the superficial or more usually the deep system because of intraluminal (thrombosis) or extraluminal (compression by tumour or other mass) obstruction is the commonest cause. However, lymphatic agenesis or obstruction causes chronic swelling. Systemic conditions — heart or renal failure — may lie behind diffuse symmetrical oedema. Lower limb swelling of all causes is aggravated by gravity. Non-invasive assessment, particularly with ultrasound (duplex, colour-duplex), is very useful in differentiating potentially lethal problems such as deep venous thrombosis from less dangerous conditions not requiring urgent therapeutic intervention.

Popliteal venous entrapment (p. 170) is a rare cause of a swollen lower limb but one that should be borne in mind in that it is treatable.

Varicose veins (Chapter 5) may be a clinical feature of incompetent valves between the superficial and deep systems alone or of incompetence *within* the deep system with secondary varicosities developing because of the exposure of the superficial to deep valves to abnormally high pressures. Varicosities of either type are possibly the most common problem in a venous clinic. The clinical diagnosis is readily made in subjects with irregularly dilated, tortuous superficial veins. Symptoms are usually mild (fatigue, aching and moderate swelling, particularly in the evening) or absent and both they and any signs present are often relieved by leg elevation and may have disappeared in the morning after a night's rest. Long-standing varicosities may be associated with chronic oedema, skin pigmentation and ulceration. Such severe signs are often an indication of varicose veins secondary to disorders of the deep system. The distinction between involvement of the two systems in an individual patient who presents with varicose veins is not easy. Dynamic non-invasive tests are necessary to make a complete assessment.

Athletes with hypertrophied leg muscles often have prominent veins. The decrease in thickness of the subcutaneous tissue makes the veins appear prominent. Unless there is a serious venous incompetence these veins do not require treatment.

Varicosities appear in pregnancy in some 20% of women below 25 years of age and in a higher percentage (32%) in women above 26. They are very occasionally a clinical problem. Compression, leg elevation and reassurance are indicated more than treatment which may be needed only in case of superficial thrombophlebitis or deep venous thrombosis. Most veins disappear completely or almost completely within 3–8 months after delivery and any evaluation and treatment should be postponed until 12–18 months have elapsed since delivery.

Deep venous thrombosis (Chapter 6). Though varicose veins and their concomitant valvular insufficiency are the most usual chronic problems in the venous clinic, deep thrombosis is the most frequent acute problem of veins. In the USA each year some 600 000 patients are treated in hospital for the condition. Clinical manifestations of thrombosis are absent in many patients with the disorder. Swelling, pain, erythema, warmth, discomfort, calf tenderness, a positive Homans sign (calf pain on dorsiflexion of the ankle), fever, tachycardia and elevated sedimentation rate may be present. However, pulmonary embolism and thrombosis often occur without any signs or symptoms in the leg and are common, sometimes fatal, complications of major surgical procedures, particularly those which are followed by immobilization. Avoidance of deep vein thrombosis and its consequences involves careful education of those susceptible and prevention of the condition because treatment of the established condition is expensive and only partly effective.

Pulmonary thromboembolism (Chapter 7) is a direct consequence of venous thrombosis which may occur in any clinical setting but is most common in elderly, immobilized and very ill or injured patients. Though non-fatal episodes are three to five times as common as fatal ones, about 150 000 patients die annually from pulmonary thromboembolism in the USA and it is responsible for at least 5% of all postoperative deaths. Between a quarter and a half of postoperative deaths are in patients with an otherwise good prognosis. As mentioned above, peripheral symptoms and signs are frequently absent. There is also an increased risk of pulmonary embolism during pregnancy and the puerperium.

With a large pulmonary embolus there is a sudden onset of dyspnoea and the patient is often anxious whether or not there is chest pain. Signs of acute right heart failure and circulatory collapse may follow after a few minutes. Pulmonary infarction (regarded as a different condition from pulmonary embolism in this context) may be associated with less severe dyspnoea, pleuritic pain, cough, haemoptysis, and peripheral x-ray density in the lung. The diagnosis is suggested by ventilation/perfusion scanning but is established only by pulmonary angiography.

Superficial thrombophlebitis (Chapter 9) is often associated with a tender, indurated, palpable 'cord' along the line of a superficial (usually varicose) vein. The long saphenous vein or one of its tributaries, most often below the knee, is usually affected. Redness and heat may be observed in the affected area but usually the limb is not swollen. Rarely, deep venous thrombosis may follow if the tail of the thrombus extends into a deep vein. In about 35% of patients systemic signs (low grade fever and, rarely, an increased white cell count) may also be present. In the upper extremities self-administration of drugs or an indwelling catheter are common causes.

Subclavian and axillary venous thrombosis (SAVT) (Chapter 10) is less common than deep venous thrombosis of the legs and accounts for only 1–2% of detected cases of deep venous thrombosis. The relatively low incidence of subclavian thrombosis is thought to be due to the short length of these veins and the relative absence of venous stasis compared to the lower limbs. Swelling of the entire arm and distension of collateral veins over the anterior chest wall may be present. Swelling and pain are usually worse during exercise. Often patients describe a history of unusual effort or muscular activity of the upper extremity before the onset of the condition. Imaging may occasionally reveal obstruction of a proximal vein at the thoracic outlet.

Chronic venous insufficiency (CVI) (Chapter 11) is the descriptive term for the changes which develop—almost exclusively in the lower limb—when there is an increase in venous pressure in both deep and superficial veins consequent upon valve damage with reflux and/or obstruction to outflow. It is a widespread, serious and often underestimated problem affecting some 0.5% of the populations of the UK and USA and some 0.31% in Italy. It has been calculated that two million workdays are lost in the USA each year because of complications caused by CVI. Most cases are, or are considered to be, late sequelae of deep venous thrombosis, hence the term *postphlebitic syndrome*, generally used to define (not always correctly) CVI. Other factors, such as congenital absence or incompetence of the valves, congenital or chronic dilatation of the deep or superficial venous system, may be the initiating cause. However, the usual antecedent is a deep vein thrombosis but a history of such a clinical episode is often absent. Chronic oedema, hyperpigmentation, skin induration and lipodermatosclerosis (see p. 126) of the distal leg and ankle are associated with the chronically increased venous pressure. Secondary varicose veins may be present. A chronic increase in venous pressure is the outcome of reflux in the deep and/or the superficial system and/or of some degree of obstruction. In the most severe cases, obstruction and reflux are associated. Ulceration, especially above the medial malleolus, is the final outcome in CVI.

Venous ulcerations are a complex, expensive problem, difficult to manage and with many social implications. Most often the problem is not only the purely clinical one of the severity of the venous disorder but includes other factors such as lack of care of the original venous problem, immobility and stasis often associated with obesity and old people living alone who are incapable of taking care of themselves. It is important to differentiate a vascular, often venous, problem which requires appropriate treatment from the social problem. Many of these patients have limited venous incompetence or no venous problem at all and what they require is advice, mobilization and daily care by a nurse or members of their family.

Lymphoedema (Chapter 12) is the consequence of an abnormal collection of interstitial lymph fluid because of poor lymphatic drainage, as distinct from an increased venous pressure. Insufficient numbers of lymphatic channels may be present because of a congenital developmental abnormality; alternatively, secondary lymphatic obstruction may develop as, for example, after destruction of lymphatic channels by radiation or filarial inflammation. Progressive swelling of one or both lower extremities, often without antecedent history, is observed. Non-pitting oedema is usually present and recurrent episodes of **lymphangitis** and cellulitis may occur. The oedema does not respond to elevation.

Other common venous problems caused by incompetence or high pressure in the venous system are the following:

Haemorrhoids (Chapter 13), dilatation of the plexus of haemorrhoidal veins and enlargement of the anal cushions, are associated with bleeding, protrusion, discomfort and severe pain and may cause anaemia.

Varicocele (Chapter 13) is the outcome of incompetence of valves in the spermatic and testicular veins. Tortuosity and dilatation of the pampiniform plexus is seen and may be associated with male infertility.

Pelvic congestion syndrome (Chapter 13), a less common (or probably only more difficult to diagnose) problem, involves the pelvic and ovarian veins and is characterized by pelvic pain and pelvic venous abnormalities (ovarian vein reflux, vulvar varices).

Venous trauma, acquired arteriovenous fistulas (Chapter 14) and **tumours involving the veins** (i.e. the inferior or superior vena cava) are conditions which usually require specialized investigation and prompt treatment should always be in the mind of the clinician in that they may occasionally be confused with other causes of venous obstruction (e.g. thrombosis).

RARE VENOUS PROBLEMS (Chapter 14)

The Klippel–Trenaunay syndrome (KTS) consists of a complex of vascular anomalies mainly involving arteriovenous fistulas usually present at birth which develop further with growth. Clinical presentation is varied and considered in detail on p. 162.

Congenital arteriovenous communications (fistulas) In the congenital diffuse type, small precapillary arteriovenous communications are present and usually cannot be detected by angiography. The affected limb may be warmer and grow faster. In some cases haemangiomatous changes may be associated but often there is no venous component.

Haemangiomas   At a very early stage in angiogenesis before arteries, veins and lymphatics become separately identifiable, vessels contain all three vascular elements. Localized haemangiomas are a persistence of this state after birth, usually with a prevalence of the venous component and are of two types: capillary and cavernous. Their management is considered on p. 164.

Renal venous thrombosis (RVT) in newborns and adults is usually unilateral but may be bilateral. It is a complex condition which requires specialized investigation and management.

OBSTRUCTION OF THE VENAE CAVA (p. 170)

Inferior vena cava   Extension of a renal carcinoma into the renal vein and then the cava may cause high obstruction. Other causes are lymph node masses in the retroperitoneum and thrombosis secondary to systemic disease.

Table 3.1 Venous and lymphatic diseases

Swollen limb (15%)
Varicose veins (27%)
Deep venous thrombosis (18%)
Pulmonary thromboembolism (0.5%)
Superficial thrombophlebitis (6%)
Subclavian/axillary venous thrombosis (1%)
Chronic venous insufficiency and postphlebitic syndrome (22%)
Lymphoedema (3%)
Varicocele (9%)
Pelvic congestion syndrome (0.5%)
Venous trauma (0.2%)
Arteriovenous communications and fistulas (0.7%)
Tumours involving the veins (0.1%)
Athletes' prominent veins (0.5%)
Dilated and varicose veins in pregnancy (1%)
Venous ulcerations (12%)
Rare problems (1.2%)
  Renal vein thrombosis
    newborns
    adults
  Popliteal vein entrapment
  Renal adenocarcinoma extending into the inferior vena cava
Congenital venous anomalies (1.3%)
  Klippel–Trenaunay syndrome
  Haemangiomas
    capillary
    cavernous
Splenic vein thrombosis (0.1%)

Note: The patients' distribution reflects several factors and may be variable from place to place on the basis of the interest and service offered by the venous clinic and on the type of referrals (i.e. the availability of all range of non-invasive vascular tests). The actual prevalence of these diseases in the general population in clinical form or in a subclinical phase is unknown. The San Valentino project in Central Italy aims to establish the actual prevalence of all ranges of vascular (arterial and venous diseases) in the entire population of a single village. The study includes a complete non-invasive assessment in the analysis of symptomatic and asymptomatic subjects.

Superior vena cava Malignant disease in the superior mediastinum is the most common cause but disorders of clotting and the use of indwelling catheters are other causes.

Splenic and portal disorders (portal hypertension, hepatic and splenic vein thrombosis) are, with the exception of the last, not considered in this book as these problems are usually associated with complex gastrointestinal and hepatic disease.

Table **3.1** summarizes the spectrum of venous diseases in a sample of 10 000 patients seen in a single clinic and indicates the percentage of patients with each problem after full diagnostic assessment. In 20% of these patients more than one problem was present.

CHAPTER 4

Assessment of the venous and lymphatic systems

VENOUS SYSTEM AND VENOUS INSUFFICIENCY

GENERAL CONSIDERATIONS

Venous insufficiency has been defined (p. 13) as the changes which develop—almost exclusively in the lower limb—when there is an increase in venous pressure in either the superficial veins alone or both the deep and superficial veins consequent upon valve damage with reflux from the deep to superficial system and/or obstruction to outflow. The term *chronic* is used when these changes are of some standing and produce effects on the dynamics of the venous system and on the nutrition of the skin and subcutaneous tissues.

The first objective is to detect whether obstruction or reflux is present. Second, the anatomical localization of the abnormality must be found. Finally, the problem of quantification of the reflux or obstruction must be addressed. These objectives can, to a great extent, be achieved by non-invasive methods though invasive techniques may be needed in some complex circumstances.

NON-INVASIVE METHODS

In evaluating CVI, non-invasive tests combine physiological and imaging techniques. For the most part, these tests are widely available, simple, quick and cost-effective. Therefore, they are the methods of choice for initial objective evaluation as distinct from clinical diagnosis.

The latest advances and current thinking indicate that the optimum useful information can be obtained using only three instruments:

- ◆ pocket Doppler;
- ◆ duplex scanning device, preferably with colour-flow imaging;
- ◆ air plethysmography.

A pocket Doppler is a simple ultrasound instrument generally used without any form of chart recording for rapid evaluation of arterial and venous flow velocity. The qualitative assessment obtained with a pocket Doppler usually indicates the presence or absence of arterial and venous flow (easily separating the two) and some limited characteristics of the flow (phasicity with respiration, etc.). This instrument can be used with excellent results even by subjects with limited experience in ultrasound. Duplex scanners combine B-mode ultrasound imaging and pulsed Doppler which may be focused on the part of the image (i.e. the artery or vein) to be evaluated. A more precise selective flow velocity evaluation is possible with duplex at the expense of time and cost increase. Usually some experience is needed to use these instruments. The more sophisticated colour-coded duplex scanner systems are more expensive and complex and require a wider knowledge of technology to be fully used. They are not used (as the pocket Doppler) quickly to assess outpatients or patients in the ward.

Tests for venous reflux

Venous reflux is generally the result of gravity or of an increase in abdominal pressure directing venous blood distally. Therefore, reflux testing should be performed with the patient standing. Recent studies have shown that venous reflux detected while examining the venous system with duplex when a subject is in the supine position is frequently abolished when the patient is standing. This is because closure of valve cusps occurs only after venous reflux exceeds a critical flow velocity, causing the valve cusps to move and close.

This is achieved with the patient standing rather than supine. When the patient is standing, it is important that muscular contractions are avoided. Therefore, the patient should be examined holding onto a frame or table. The leg to be examined should be relaxed, with the knee slightly flexed and the weight on the opposite leg, because it has been shown that, during full knee extension, an occlusion of the popliteal vein occurs in 20% of healthy people.

After the **clinical examination**, a **pocket Doppler** instrument is used and this complements physical examination as a screening test for outpatients to evaluate the presence of the most obvious venous problems (i.e. presence of venous flow, reflux at the most important junctions such as the saphenofemoral and saphenopopliteal junctions).

The knee of the leg to be examined should be slightly flexed to relax the muscles and skin over the popliteal fossa. With the probe placed over the femoral (or popliteal) veins, muscles are manually compressed and then compression is released. Abolition of the reflux by compression of the superficial veins just below the probe (i.e. at the level of the proximal end of the long saphenous or short saphenous veins) suggests that reflux is confined to the superficial system. Failure to abolish reflux by such a manoeuvre indicates that the reflux is in the deep system (femoral or popliteal veins).

In experienced hands, the pocket Doppler provides in most patients clear answers regarding the presence or absence of reflux at the saphenofemoral and/or saphenopopliteal junctions. Abnormal anatomy in the popliteal fossa is responsible for most of the errors (8%). For example, reflux in the gastrocnemius veins may be interpreted as reflux in the popliteal vein.

Also, continuous-wave Doppler is not accurate in localizing incompetent perforating veins.

Duplex and colour-duplex scanning are more effective and quicker than examination with pocket Doppler. Duplex scanning provides information about reflux in specific veins. For example, the femoral, popliteal, deep calf veins and perforating veins can be individually tested. The use of colour has made duplex scanning faster and more accurate.

As in examination of a patient with the continuous-wave instrument, the patient is examined standing (**Figures 4.1a** and **4.1b**). The lower extremity that is not bearing weight is evaluated and the sites to be studied are tested with a 5 or 7.5 MHz probe. The saphenofemoral junction (**Figure 4.1a**), the popliteal venous anatomy, the saphenopopliteal junction (**Figure 4.1b**) and the perforating

Figure 4.1
(a) Evaluation of the saphenofemoral junction with colour-duplex. The patient is standing and the weight is on the opposite limb.
(b) Evaluation of the veins in the popliteal space.

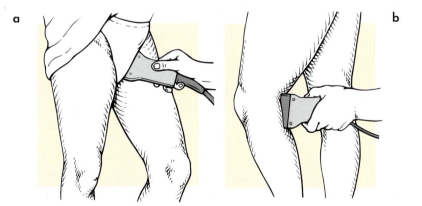

Figure 4.2 (a) Flow in the saphenofemoral junction is shown during a manual compression-release manoeuvre of the thigh. Blue colour on calf compression indicates cephalad flow. (b) Reflux is indicated by red colour on release of the compression. Reflux (red) at the saphenofemoral junction and in the proximal section of the saphenous vein, lasting for more than 1 second after release of manual compression indicates incompetence.

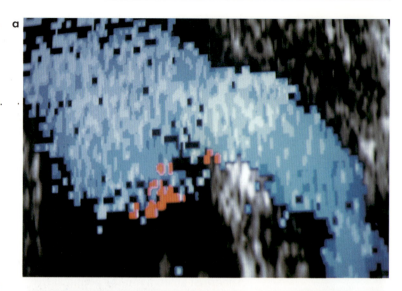

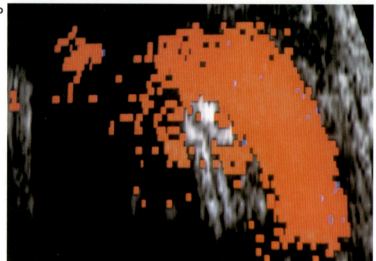

veins are successively visualized. Manual calf compression or, ideally, compression by a rapidly deflatable cuff is used. The cuff inflation produces cephalad flow (blue in **Figure 4.2a**). Rapid release of the compression is essential in testing for reflux (red in **Figure 4.2b**) or to show competence (absent reflux) or valve closure. **Figures 4.3a** and **4.3b** show the saphenopopliteal junction and the veins in the popliteal fossa.

In chronic venous insufficiency causing ulceration (**Figure 4.4**) the localization of the perforating veins which are associated with venous hypertension may be very important. **Figure 4.5** shows diagrammatically an example of testing for perforating veins. The corresponding colour-duplex image is in **Figure 4.6**. Localization of

Figure 4.3
(a) Detection of reflux at the saphenopopliteal junction with manual compression of the calf.
(b) Three different but common anatomical variations of the veins in the popliteal fossa are shown. Colour-duplex scanning reveals the anatomy and enables testing of each individual vein for reflux.

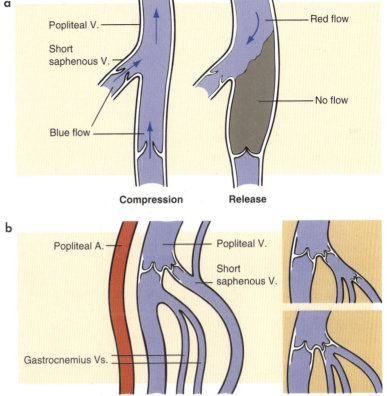

Figure 4.4 Area of venous hypertension with initial ulceration. The high venous pressure is associated with the presence of a large, incompetent perforating vein close to the ulceration.

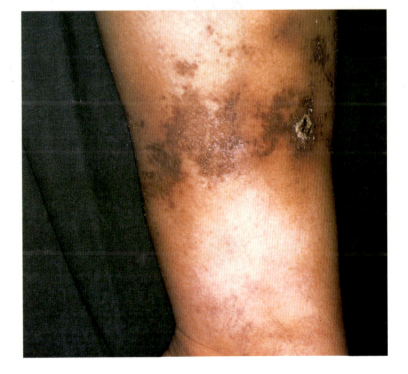

Figure 4.5 Transverse scan of superficial and deep veins. (a) By moving the probe up or down the limb with continuous visualization of the two veins the presence and level of a communicating vein are determined. (b) The direction of flow with calf compression and release can then be tested.

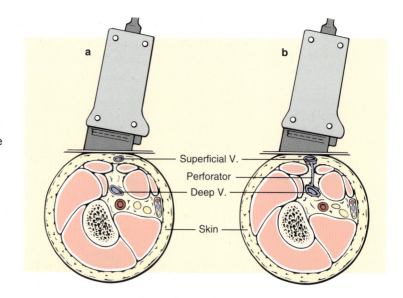

Superficial V.
Perforator
Deep V.
Skin

Figure 4.6 A large, incompetent perforating vein close to the ulceration shown in Figure 4.4.

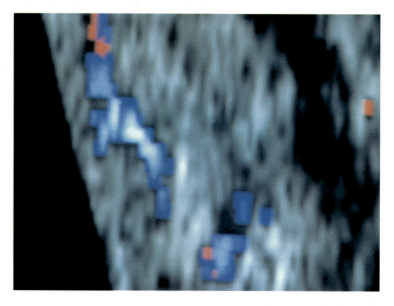

calf perforating veins and reflux through them is time-consuming with conventional duplex but colour-flow imaging has made this test practical.

Colour-duplex scanning for localization of sites of reflux is particularly useful in patients with recurrent varicose veins after previous surgery. Such examination also confirms normal function in deep veins and the extent and site of venous reflux when it is present. Both localized and generalized reflux—that is, reflux present throughout the deep venous system—can be identified.

Qualification of reflux in individual veins is possible but very time-consuming. Accurate and reproducible results are obtained easily for the whole leg using air plethysmography, which has become the test of choice for quantitating reflux (see p. 40).

Ambulatory venous pressure

The minimally invasive measurement of venous pressure is a standard with which other examinations are compared. Venous pressure is measured by inserting a needle in a vein on the dorsum of the foot with the patient standing (**Figure 4.7**). Pressures are recorded during a ten tiptoe exercise test and the ambulatory venous pressure (AVP) is defined as the lowest pressure reached during the exercise. AVP is a function of a calf muscle pump ejection capacity, the magnitude of reflux and the outflow resistance. Therefore, it represents the net effect of all the abnormalities that affect venous haemodynamics. In normal limbs, the AVP is less than 30 mmHg (clinical measurements are indicated in mmHg) and the refilling time (RT) is longer than 18 seconds. These values are the consequence of filling of the veins from the arterial side. When venous reflux (superficial and/or deep) is present, the AVP tends to be higher (i.e. above 40–50 mmHg) and the refilling time is shortened (**Table 4.1**). After AVP has been measured, the exercise test is repeated with narrow tourniquets (2.5 cm wide) applied at the ankle, below the knee, and in the thigh.

Figure 4.7 Recording of venous pressure during ten tiptoe exercises with and without a below-knee cuff (2.5 cm wide) that occluded the superficial veins. Normal values for ambulatory venous pressure (P) and RT_{90} indicate that the valves of the deep veins are competent.

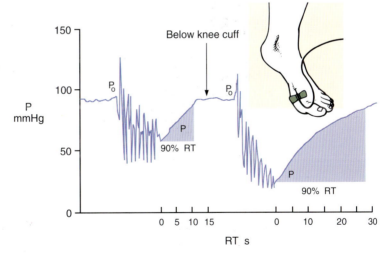

These tourniquets control reflux from the superficial veins and if superficial reflux is present, the AVP and RT are returned to normal values. In patients with incompetence in the deep veins, this does not occur. Table 4.1 indicates that AVP is higher than normal in the presence of venous reflux at the saphenopopliteal valve. For AVPs of 40–100 mmHg, there is a linear relationship with the incidence of skin ulceration. This is true regardless of the underlying cause and whether the incompetence is in the superficial or the deep system (**Table 4.1**).

Photoplethysmography (PPG) and light reflection rheography (LRR)

In an attempt to obtain RT by non-invasive means, PPG and LRR tests were devised. In both of these techniques, a photodetector is applied to the skin of the foot or ankle (**Figure 4.8**). These methods, using the reflection of infrared light into the skin, are based on the concept that the presence of increased venous blood in the superficial skin capillaries affects light transmission and reflection. These techniques (PPG and LRR are broadly comparable) were developed to detect whether incompetence of the venous system is mainly superficial or deep.

Figure 4.8
Measurement of RT or RT_{90} using photoplethysmography.

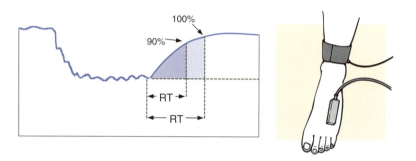

Table 4.1 Ambulatory venous pressure (AVP) and refilling time (RT)*

	AVP (mmHg)		RT_{90} (s)	
Type of limb	No ankle cuff	Ankle cuff	No ankle cuff	Ankle cuff
Normal	15–30	15–30	18–40	18–40
Primary varicose veins with competent perforating veins	25–40	15–30	10–18	18–35
Primary varicose veins with incompetent perforating veins	40–70	25–60[†]	5–15	8–30
Deep venous reflux (incompetent popliteal valves)	55–85	50–80	3–15	5–15
Popliteal reflux and proximal occlusion	60–110	60–120		
Popliteal occlusion and competent popliteal valves	25–60	10–60		

* Standard exercise: 10 tiptoe movements.
† In one-third of these limbs, AVP remained more than 40 mmHg and RT_{90} less than 15 seconds despite the application of the ankle cuff.

Table 4.2 shows the PPG refilling times with or without an ankle cuff in position, in normal controls, in patients with superficial reflux and in those with deep venous incompetence. Better reproducibility and better separation of groups can be obtained when the test is performed with the patient upright.

It should be emphasized that both RT and RT_{90} (the time taken for 90% of filling to take place) obtained with PPG or LRR are poor measures of the severity of deep venous disease. In patients with chronic venous incompetence (i.e. due to popliteal vein incompetence), a clinically significant reduction in AVP from 100 to 60 mmHg, produced by a successful venous valve substitution or valvuloplasty, thus has little effect on the RT_{90} obtained with PPG or LLR. Therefore, these methods are not suitable to assess and quantify the effects of reconstructive venous surgery but only as screening methods to evaluate whether patients have venous insufficiency, whether this is mainly superficial or deep and expressing the degree of insufficiency in a semiquantitative scale (seconds of refilling time).

Air plethysmography
(APG)

APG uses a calibrated air chamber applied to encompass a leg (**Figure 4.9**). A detailed technical description of the method is beyond the scope of this book. In simple terms, plethysmography methods such as strain gauge or air plethysmography are based on the electronic detection of small volumetric changes in a limb. Air plethysmography provides quantitative information about the various components of the calf muscle pump. These include:

◆ rate of filling of the venous reservoir (venous filling index, VFI) as a result of standing, namely the variation in volume produced in a limb in a defined time by the passage from the supine to the

Figure 4.9 Diagram of the air plethysmograph. The 100 ml syringe included in the circuit is used for calibration.

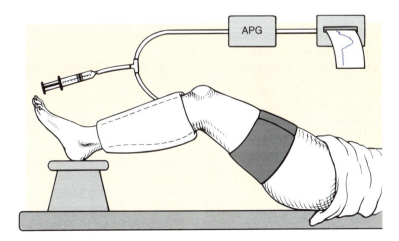

Table 4.2 Photoplethysmographic refilling time (RT_{90}) with and without an ankle cuff to occlude superficial veins

	Standing (s)		Sitting (s)	
	No cuff	Cuff	No cuff	Cuff
Normal	18 – 80*	18 – 80	26 – 100	26 – 100
SVI	5 – 18	18 – 50	2 – 25	18 – 50
DVI	3 – 12	6 – 18†	2 – 28	2 – 30

* RT_{90} > 18 seconds without cuff identifies normal limbs.

† RT_{90} < 18 seconds with cuff identifies limbs with deep venous incompetence.

Table 4.3 Air plethysmography

Direct measurements	Units	Coefficient of variation	Normal limbs	Primary VVs	DVD
Functional venous volume (VV) (increase in leg volume on standing)	ml	10.8 – 12.5	100 – 150	100 – 350	70 – 320
Venous filling time (VFT_{90}) (time taken to reach 90% of VV)	s	8.0 – 11.5	70 – 170	5 – 70	5 – 20
Ejected volume (EV) (decrease in leg volume as a result of one tiptoe)	ml	6.7 – 9.4	60 – 150	50 – 180	8 – 140
Residual volume (RV) (volume of blood left in veins after ten tiptoes)	ml	6.2 – 12	2 – 45	50 – 150	60 – 200
Derived measurements					
Venous filling index (VFI) (average filling rate 90% VF/VFT_{90})	ml/s	5.3 – 8	0.5 – 1.7	2 – 25	7 – 30
Ejection fraction (EF = [EV/VV] x 100)	%	2.9 – 9.5	60 – 90	25 – 70	20 – 50
Residual volume fraction (RVF = [RV/VV] x 100)	%	4.3 – 8.2	2 – 35	25 – 80	30 – 100

VVs, varicose veins; DVD, deep venous disease

Figure 4.10
The manoeuvres and methods of deriving the air plethysmographic measurements.

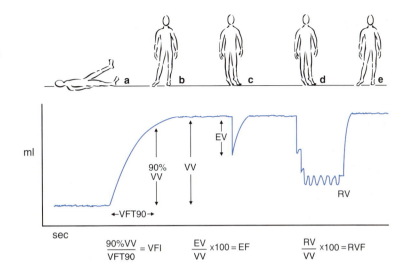

$$\frac{90\%VV}{VFT90} = VFI \qquad \frac{EV}{VV} \times 100 = EF \qquad \frac{RV}{VV} \times 100 = RVF$$

standing position (this volume is low in normal limbs and increased between 3 to 5 times in chronic venous disease and large varicose veins);
◆ venous volume (VV), which is the amount of blood in the venous reservoir;
◆ ejected volume (EV) and the ejection fraction (EF = [EV/VV] x 100) as a result of a single step;
◆ residual volume (RV) and residual volume fraction (RVF = [RV/VV] x 100) as a result of ten tiptoe movements.

The manoeuvres and methods of making these measurements from the recording are shown diagrammatically in **Figure 4.10**.

There is a high reproducibility of measurements expressed as ratios: VFI, EF and RVF all have a coefficient of variation less than 10% (**Table 4.3**). VFI is a measurement of the quantity of refluxing venous blood in the limb and is expressed as ml/s. The median and 90% range of the various measurements in different

Table 4.4 Incidence of ulceration in relation to ambulatory venous pressure (AVP) in 222 patients (251 limbs)

AVP (mmHg)	No.	Incidence of ulceration
<30	34	0
30–40	44	11
41–50	51	22
51–60	45	38
61–70	34	59
71–80	28	68
81–90	10	60
>90	5	100

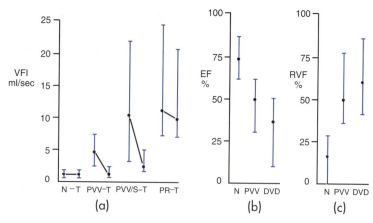

Figure 4.11 (a) Venous filling time (VFI) in normal controls, in limbs with primary varicose veins without (PVV) and with skin changes (PVV/S) and limbs with popliteal reflux (PR). The results are presented as median and 90% range without and with a 2.5 cm tourniquet (T) at the knee that occluded the superficial veins. The application of this tourniquet can differentiate between reflux in the superficial and deep veins. (b) Ejection fraction (EF) in normal controls, limbs with primary varicose veins (PVV) and deep venous disease (DVD). The results are presented as median and 90% range. (c) Residual volume fraction (RVF) in the same group of patients as in (a) and (b).

groups of patients are shown in **Figure 4.11** (a), (b) and (c) and in Table 4.3.

The linear correlation that exists between RVF and the AVP (**Figure 4.12**) indicates that an estimate of the AVP can be obtained non-invasively from the RVF.

The incidence of cutaneous ulceration increases with increase in AVP (Table 4.4), and amount of reflux (VFI), and a decrease in the efficiency of the calf muscle pump ejection (EF). Thus, the RFV provides information on the overall effect of all the venous abnormalities. In addition, the abnormalities are dissected out and measured in terms of the EF (ejection) and the VFI (reflux) components.

Tests for outflow obstruction

Ascending venography (see p. 46) remains the standard method of delineating persistent obstruction to venous return. However, there are several non-invasive tests that determine the presence and quantify the degree of obstruction to outflow from the lower limb. Simple continuous-wave Doppler measurement can be used as a screening device in outpatients. A history of deep thrombosis or

Figure 4.12 Correlation between AVP and RVF.

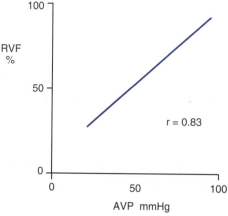

persistent leg and ankle swelling suggests the need for such an examination.

Although not yet in general use, the best test to evaluate obstruction is the arm–foot pressure differential developed by Raju (see below).

Other non-invasive tests are based on the measurements of venous outflow by various techniques and using different instrumentation. These methods include the strain-gauge, impedance and air plethysmography modalities. Most tests are now mainly used world wide for clinical research applications or for clinical evaluation in specialized centres interested in venous physiology and surgery. It is important to observe that different protocols of evaluation are available and a consensus has not been reached yet on the clinical applications of these methods. Our opinion is that the high reproducibility and simplicity of air plethysmography has made this technique the method of choice; however, other methods are in more general use.

Ultrasound techniques: continuous-wave Doppler and duplex scanning

The patient is examined with the legs horizontal and the knee slightly flexed. The trunk should be at 45 degrees and the ultrasound probe is held over the femoral vein. Flow velocity is normally phasic with respiration and if this is established a normal iliac segment is present. Absence of phasic flow or the finding of flow that is continuous and not affected by respirations suggests obstruction. If flow is diminished or abolished by compression of the contralateral groin or suprapubic area, the presence of obstruction and a collateral circulation is established. Augmentation of the velocity of blood in the common femoral vein by calf compression indicates absence of popliteal and femoral venous obstruction. This manoeuvre can be repeated with occlusion by external pressure of the long saphenous vein at the knee which provides a double check on the patency of the popliteal vein. Augmentation of the velocity in the popliteal vein produced by gentle compression of each muscular compartment of the leg draining into the branches of the popliteal vein suggests that the relative venous branch is patent.

Duplex and colour-duplex imaging detect with great accuracy the particular veins which contain organized thrombus and which are in consequence not compressible by pressure from the probe. Such duplex visualization of the deep veins may even reveal irregular vein walls with abnormal echo and a partially recanalized lumen.

Arm – foot pressure differential

The arm–foot pressure differential measurement is considered to be an excellent method of quantitating outflow obstruction. The technique is to record the venous pressure in the veins of the foot

Table 4.5 Arm–foot differential in limbs with outflow obstruction.

Grade	Pressure at rest (mmHg)	Pressure increment during hyperaemia
I Fully compensated	<5	<6
II Partially compensated	<5	<6
III Partially decompensated	>5	>6 (often 10–15)
IV Fully decompensated	>>>5	No further increase (often 15–20)

and hand simultaneously after venous cannulation. The measurements are made with the patient supine and are repeated after inducing reactive hyperaemia in the leg.

The normal arm–foot pressure differential is less than 5 mmHg with a rise of 1–6 mmHg (i.e. 5 may rise by 1–6 mmHg, to become 6–11 mmHg) during reactive hyperaemia. Patients with venographically proven evidence of obstruction have been classified into four grades according to the criteria shown in **Table 4.5**.

Outflow measurements

The degree of venous obstruction can be assessed from outflow measurements using a mercury strain-gauge or air plethysmography. In both techniques, a proximal thigh cuff is inflated to a pressure sufficient to occlude the venous system (i.e. 100–120 mmHg) with the patient supine and the limb elevated by 10 degrees with external rotation and 10 degrees of knee flexion. The veins are allowed to fill for at least 2 minutes and the cuff is suddenly deflated. The following measurements are made from the outflow curves: maximum venous outflow; 1-second outflow; and 3-second outflow. All are valid measurements used and advocated by different authors. The outflow fraction is expressed as

$$OF = (V_1/VV) \times 100$$

Table 4.6 shows the range of values for limbs with normal veins, moderate, and severe obstruction measured by strain gauge (MVO) and air plethysmography (OF). The correlation between outflow fraction using air plethysmography and arm–foot pressure differentials is good ($r > 0.7$); for outflow resistance it can be calculated from the APG and direct venous pressure outflow curves obtained simultaneously (**Figure 4.13**).

Outflow (Q) can be calculated from the tangent at any point on the volume outflow curve. Resistance (R) is calculated by dividing the corresponding pressure (P) by the flow (Q):

$$R = P/Q$$

Table 4.6 Maximum venous outflow (MVO)

Obstruction	Normal	Moderate	Severe
MVO strain-gauge (1 s) (ml/100 ml per min)	14	45 – 30	30
1 sec outflow fraction (OF) air plethysmography (% of VV)	38	38 – 30	30

VV, venous volume.

Figure 4.13 Pressure and volume inflow and outflow curves obtained simultaneously using an APG and cannulation of a vein on the dorsum of the foot.

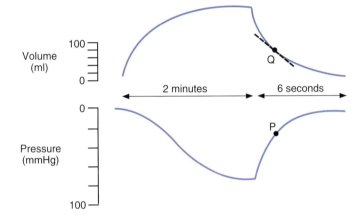

Figure 4.14 Relation between outflow resistance curves and Raju classification of outflow obstruction (grades I–IV) (N, normal limbs).

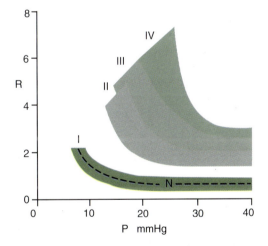

This can be done for a series of points on the outflow curves. Plotting the resistance against the pressure (**Figure 4.13**), produces a non-linear relation. At low pressures, when the veins are collapsed, the resistance is high but decreases as the pressure rises, presumably with increased venous distension.

Figure 4.14 demonstrates the relationship between the resistance and the four grades of arm–foot pressure differential described by Raju.

To **conclude**, it is now possible to detect the presence or absence of reflux or obstruction in venous circulation non-invasively, define the anatomical site and obtain quantitative measures of the severity of both.

Optimum information can be obtained using simple tools such as a pocket Doppler, duplex and colour-duplex scanning and APG.

THE ROLE OF INVASIVE TESTING OF MORPHOLOGY AND FUNCTION

For patients who would be candidates for reconstructive surgery, further knowledge of morphology and function is necessary after the non-invasive testing. We have to differentiate between venous obstruction and reflux and whether the reflux is due to primary valve incompetence with reparable deep valves from post-thrombotic patients with destroyed valves. In obstruction we need to search out pathways for various bypasses in the iliac or rarely the femoral veins. In iliac obstruction ascending and descending phlebography combined with femoral venous pressure measurements are the invasive methods of choice.

Ascending phlebography

Ascending phlebography is important in all candidates for deep reconstruction and most of the candidates for perforators surgery. Ascending phlebography is useful in patients with chronic venous insufficiency to map the patient's veins in the extremities and to identify the incompetent perforating veins in the calf. It will also identify obstructed venous segments in the calf, thigh and pelvis and most of the recanalized post-thrombotic segments. Ascending phlebography will also provide a map of patent veins in the extremity.

Descending phlebography

Descending phlebography is necessary to plan a deep vein valve reconstruction or valve substitution procedures and is the only reliable means to differentiate primary valve incompetence (PVI) from secondary, post-thrombotic valve incompetence (SVI) as a cause of deep vein reflux in the proximal thigh. Individual study of the long saphenous vein, superficial femoral vein and profunda femoral vein is done to identify the presence of valves and their state of competence with and without Valsalva.

When reflux occurs through a proximal valve the contrast is followed distally in that segment until it dissipates. The descending phlebogram is interpreted, considering the distal extent of reflux.

When reflux is limited to the thigh veins the patient is not considered to be a candidate for deep vein valve surgery. When reflux passes through the popliteal vein and into the calf, surgical correction is deemed appropriate. Because the descending phlebogram is a dynamic study, it is necessary to perform the test under fluoroscopy and it is important to record a videotape of the study for future analysis.

In patients with iliac vein obstruction the functional importance of the obstruction should be evaluated at the time of femoral phlebography.

Bilateral femoral pressure measurements should be performed, utilizing the cannulas, in the supine, resting position and during dorsovolar flexion.

The most important indicators of functional obstruction of the iliac veins are the pressure elevation after exercise, pressure difference after exercise and pressure normalization time after exercise.

LYMPHATIC ASSESSMENT

Lymphangiography Lymphangiography is performed less often than venography or arteriography because the method may be difficult and some complications are possible. Tests of pulmonary function before lymphangiography is undertaken are advisable because the contrast medium used for lymphangiography may produce a temporary diffusion barrier when it reaches the lungs.

Method An organic dye (i.e. methylene blue) is injected into the skin and passes via the subdermal or superficial dermal lymphatic system into the local lymphatics. A channel can then be seen and exposed for cannulation and direct injection of contrast medium. The radiographic lymphangiogram obtained usually shows lymphatics of uniform diameter branching as they approach the proximal part of the limb. The technique is helpful in detecting the cause of chronic swelling of the limbs and differentiating primary from secondary lymphoedema (Chapter 12). Lymphangiography is also used (but this is fairly uncommon nowadays) to study lymph nodes in the retroperitoneum and mediastinum in the evaluation of patients with lymphomas.

Lymphoscintigraphy This relatively simple test, which is without important side effects, is usually performed on an outpatient basis (**Figure 4.15**).

Figure 4.15 (a) ^{99}Tc lymphoscintigraphy (early scan) shows a dilatation of the lymphatics (right side of the picture). (b) A late scan shows presence of the isotope at the contralateral thigh, with low captation of the affected limb (right side of picture).

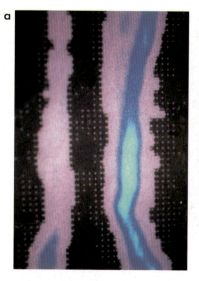
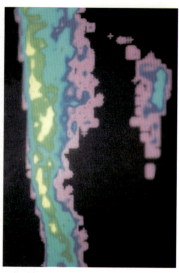

Method

After injection of a small amount of technetium-99 m labelled antimony trisulphide colloid into an interdigital space, the extremity is imaged with a gamma camera. The movement of lymph into the lymphatics can be followed anatomically. The *appearance time* of the colloid in the regional lymph nodes indicates whether lymphatic flow and channels are normal or abnormal. In lymphoedema there are abnormal patterns with delayed appearance of colloid proximally. In patients with early chronic venous insufficiency and oedema, a normal or moderately increased lymph flow may be seen while in the late stages of venous insufficiency an impairment in lymphatic drainage may be encountered which is important in aggravating the clinical picture.

Other tests of lymphatic function

With the use of *high resolution B-mode imaging* of the subcutaneous tissues, dilated (echolucent) spaces are almost always found in lymphoedema that has been demonstrated by lymphangiography and lymphoscintigraphy. This simple test (**Figure 4.16**) is easy and repeatable and may be used to evaluate the progression of the disease or the effects of treatment. In the natural history of primary lymphoedema these spaces are almost always initially present only over the dorsum of the foot but then progressively extend. They are also seen less often and less diffusely in other clinical situations associated with oedema. MR scans can also demonstrate their presence.

The *spontaneous clearance of an haematoma* (**Figure 4.17**) can be assessed by injecting a small amount of blood (0.4 ml) into the subcutaneous tissue of the dorsum or lateral side of the foot. Repeated photography records the time of disappearance of the

Figure 4.16 High resolution ultrasound in a patient with lymphoedema. There are dilated interstitial spaces distally, (a) above, at the dorsum of the foot and (b) at the proximal ankle.

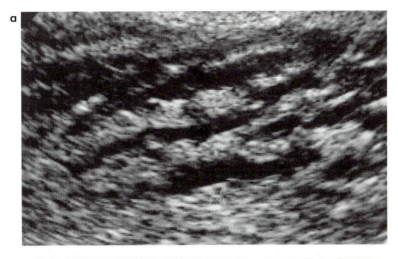

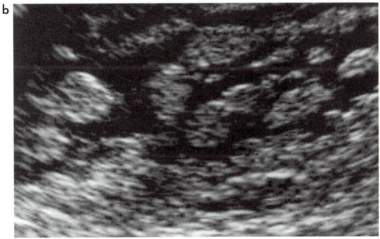

Figure 4.17 Spontaneous clearance of a small haematoma in the foot. In patients with lymphatic problems or severe post-phlebitic limbs, the surface area of the haematoma decreases more slowly than in normal subjects.

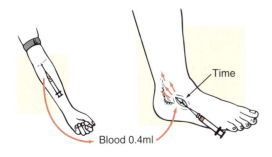

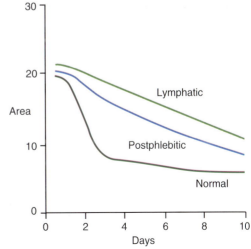

Figure 4.18
The ratio between the concentration of interstitial (lymphatic) fluid proteins and plasma proteins increases in patients with lymphatic problems and in severe chronic venous insufficiency.

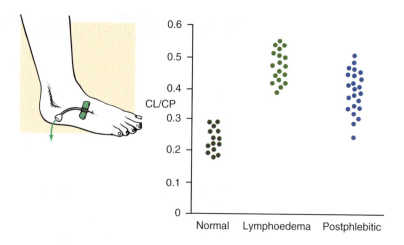

haematoma and indirectly the activity of the lymphatic system. While in normal subjects the haematoma disappears in 24–48 hours, in primary lymphoedema the disappearance time is prolonged (i.e. 3–6 days).

The *ratio between the concentation of interstitial (lymphatic) fluid and the concentration of plasma proteins* can also be assessed by obtaining a sample of interstitial fluid with a fine gauge needle inserted into the subcutaneous tissue of the dorsum of the foot (10 minutes) while the patient is resting supine. A blood sample is also taken to evaluate the plasma protein concentration. In patients with lymphatic problems an increased concentration of macromolecules (proteins) is usually observed because of the decreased lymphatic drainage (the normal ratio and the ratio in patients is shown in **Figure 4.18**). In late chronic venous insufficiency the drainage of proteins from the interstitial space may also be impaired (**Figure 4.18**).

Direct measurement of lymphatic pressure has indicated an increased pressure in patients with lymphoedema.

Except for high resolution ultrasound (which still has to be validated), these investigation methods are mainly used for research and are not easily available in most hospitals.

BIBLIOGRAPHY

Belcaro G, Christopoulos D, Nicolaides AN. Venous insufficiency: noninvasive testing. In: Bergan J, Kistner R, eds. *Atlas of Venous Surgery.* Philadelphia, USA: Saunders, 1992: p. 9.

Bergan J, Kistner R, eds. *Atlas of Venous Surgery.* Philadelphia: Saunders, 1992: pp. 9–24.

Browse NL. The diagnosis and management of primary lymphedema. *J Vasc Surg* 1986; **3**: 181.

Cesarone MR, De Sanctis MT, Laurora G, *et al.* Linfedema: nuove metodiche non invasive per la diagnosi ed il follow up. *Min Cardioangiol* 1995; **43** (in press).

Christopoulos D, Nicolaides AN. Noninvasive diagnosis and quantitation of popliteal reflux in the swollen and ulcerated leg. *J Cardiovasc Surg* 1988; **29**: 535.

Christopoulos D, Nicolaides AN, Cook A, *et al.* Pathogenesis of venous ulceration in relation to the calf muscle pump function. *Surgery* 1989; **106**: 829.

Christopoulos D, Nicolaides AN, Szendro G. Venous reflux: quantitation and correlation with the clinical severity of chronic venous disease. *Br J Surg* 1988; **75**: 352.

Hauck G. Kapilläre Permeabilität und Mikro-Lymphdrainage. *Vasa* 1994; **23**: 93.

Mortimer P. Principles of lymphoedema management. *BLIG (British Lymphology Interest Group) Newsletter* 1990; **5**: 1.

Nicolaides AN, Hoare M, Miles CR, *et al.* Value of ambulatory venous pressure in the assessment of venous insufficiency. *Vasc Diagn Ther* 1981; **3**: 41.

Nicolaides AN, Miles C. Photoplethysmography in the assessment of venous insufficiency. *J Vasc Surg* 1986; **5**: 405.

Nicolaides AN, Zukowski AJ. The value of dynamic venous pressure measurements. *World J Surg* 1986; **10**: 919.

Pflug JJ, Knox P. Interrelationship between veins and lymphatics in chronic venous insufficiency. *Phlebology* 1987; **2**: 93.

Raju S. New approaches to the diagnosis and treatment of venous obstruction. *J Vasc Surg* 1986; **4**(1): 42.

Vasdekis SN, Clarke H, Nicolaides AN. Quantification of venous reflux by means of duplex scanning. *J Vasc Surg* 1989; **10**: 670.

Varicose veins

GENERAL CONSIDERATIONS

Varicose veins are dilated, elongated and tortuous veins in the subcutaneous tissue. The valves are incompetent so that blood flow is not predominantly in one direction (centripetal) as in normal veins but may be temporarily centrifugal, depending upon posture, venous pressure and such factors as muscular activity. Such reflux may occur when position or rate of flow are altered. Varicosities are most common in the lower extremities but they also occur in other anatomical areas: the spermatic cord (varicocele), oesophagus (oesophageal varices) and anorectum (haemorrhoids). Some 10–20% of the world population may have varicose veins in the legs. The prevalence varies according to the characteristics of the population in that less developed people living an active life and eating a diet rich in fibre appear to have varicosities less frequently. By contrast, an increased incidence of varicose veins and haemorrhoids correlates well with the low-roughage diet consumed in developed countries; furthermore, varicose veins are more frequent in patients with diverticular disease of the colon. Varicose veins are probably more common in women. Other factors associated with an increased incidence of varicose veins are parity, constricting clothing, prolonged standing, obesity and chronic treatment with oestrogens (the first generation of oral contraceptives).

Varicose veins are generally divided into two classes: *primary* and *secondary*. Primary or simple varicose veins are usually associated with a normal deep venous system while secondary varicose veins are the consequence of deep venous disease (thrombosis, compression, obstruction or, rarely, arteriovenous fistula).

Differentiating between superficial and/or deep incompetence and simple varicose veins is not easy. *The definition of varicose veins is purely a clinical one. More correctly, the patients are considered to have (on the basis of dynamic, non-invasive tests) incompetence of the veins of the superficial system or of the deep system. Therefore, varicose veins may be considered to be only an important but not a precise indicator of the sites of venous incompetence.*

The causes of primary varicose veins are still unknown. Two major hypotheses, both incompletely satisfactory, have been developed. It is possible that both may be involved in individual circumstances.

The valvular incompetence hypothesis

Valvular incompetence between the deep and superficial systems is the most important observation in primary varicosities. This factor appears to be the most important in determining the clinical course and progression of varicose veins. The fundamental abnormality is progressive, sequential incompetence of the valvular rings in the main superficial trunks and in the communicating veins. More proximal incompetent valves result in high venous pressure being applied to the more distal valves so that, over time, segmental dilatation of that venous segment and of the next distal valvular ring takes place.

The weak wall hypothesis

This suggests that a developmental weakness of the vein wall results in progressive venous dilatation even at normal venous pressures with secondary failure of competence of the dilated valvular rings. However, in only 50% of patients with varicose veins there is a positive family history though this is not a strong argument against a developmental defect. A developmental weakness may facilitate the effects of post-natal factors.

Secondary varicosities develop after either damage, obstruction, or both in the deep venous system. Damage occurs when, in the wake of a deep venous thrombosis, recanalization of the thrombosed veins may be associated with destruction of the valve cusps so that pressure in the involved segment is increased and under certain conditions flow may be temporarily reversed. The vein stretches and incompetence may develop in the valves which connect the deep and superficial systems. Obstruction of a major proximal segment such as the inferior vena cava, iliac or femoral veins may produce an important increase in venous pressure. The deep system distal to the obstruction is then exposed to an increased pressure which has two effects:

♦ dilatation of collateral channels; and
♦ deep to superficial valvular incompetence, with increased pressure in the superficial system.

Both in valvular damage and in obstruction the end result is that the superficial system dilates to give rise to secondary varicosities. Their formation is aided by the fact that these veins have only weak external support from the subcutaneous tissue in that they are superficial to the deep fascia of the leg.

In some subjects *arteriovenous fistula* may be the cause of regional varicose veins (see also p. 165). This is indicated (using Doppler) by the presence of a continuous, high velocity, venous flow (in normal veins the venous flow is phasic with respiration).

CLINICAL FEATURES AND DIAGNOSIS

Diffuse, severe varicosities and skin complications may be asymptomatic while some patients with only small varicosities may have symptoms. Frequent complaints are leg aching and heaviness, cramps, itching and swelling. Patients often complain only of the appearance of the varicosities. Symptoms often occur after prolonged standing, are more severe in the evening and are partially or completely relieved by leg elevation, a night's rest or by the use of elastic compression.

The swelling associated with primary varicose veins is mild, localized at the ankle and foot and disappears after overnight elevation of the leg. In women, signs and symptoms may be more significant in the few days just before menstruation.

Eczema, skin dryness and scaling dermatitis associated with pruritus are often observed over large varicose veins, especially distally around the ankle.

The symptoms of uncomplicated primary varicose veins are usually mild and most patients are referred for cosmetic reasons only. Varicose veins may be painful but severe pain or disability is rarely or never associated with primary varicose veins. Often they are the outcome of other problems (muscular, articular, neurological, the presence of obesity). In such circumstances it is important to make clear to patients that their symptoms will not disappear even after correct treatment of the varicose veins. Secondary varicose veins caused by chronic deep venous valvular insufficiency are often associated with some degree of obstruction and cause more severe symptoms. If the chronic venous disease is not treated or clinically controlled, it may progress to ulceration. However, the presence of a venous ulcer does not always mean that there is deep venous insufficiency. In 30–45% of instances an ulcer is the result of long-standing superficial venous incompetence and the deep system is normal. The clinical features of venous pre-ulceration and ulceration are described in Chapter 11.

A general physical examination may reveal predisposing causes of varicosities or conditions such as obesity that suggest the best course of treatment. Inspection of the legs in the standing position will indicate the localization of the varicose veins. When either oedema or obesity is present, veins may be difficult to observe but palpation and percussion along the course of the greater saphenous vein (Schwartz test) may reveal lakes of blood in dilated veins. It is good practice to mark the position of the varicose veins on a scheme of the venous system (see Appendix) for future reference because the anatomy of varicose veins may be quite variable. Photographs of the veins may be very useful for the same purpose, especially if unusual venous patterns are present.

Mild pitting ankle oedema and slight pigmentation of the skin usually indicate a moderate, long-lasting venous hypertension and the need for treatment.

Special clinical tests The *Brodie–Trendelenburg test* is used to assess the competence of the valves in the perforating veins and of those in the great saphenous system. With the patient supine, the leg is elevated to empty blood from the superficial veins. The saphenous vein is then occluded by compression in the thigh and the patient stands up. After observing the limb for 30 seconds, the compression is removed. In normal limbs gradual filling of the superficial veins occurs from below on standing and release of compression does not alter this. However, if the saphenofemoral junction is incompetent, release of the tourniquet allows reflux from the deep system; in consequence, the veins fill rapidly. Rapid filling while compression is maintained means that there are incompetent valves at more sites. The location of these can be partly achieved by placing multiple tourniquets around the leg and thigh and observing which venous segment fills. To test the short saphenous system independently it is best to control the long saphenous vein by a separate tourniquet. Palpation along and close to the superficial varices is useful to identify incompetent perforating veins which are often associated with depressions in the fascia though these may be hollowed out merely by a dilated superficial vein. Incompetent perforating veins are most frequent in the lower leg just posterior to the medial border of the tibia.

The accuracy of the clinical examination of varicose veins is limited and subjective. It is also determined by the experience of the examiner in that the variability of the patterns of distribution and of the clinical presentation make this problem quite complex.

Simple non-invasive tests are better and quicker for initial clinical decision-making. The continuous-wave pocket Doppler (see p.

32) is very useful to exclude major deep venous problems and to define the major points of incompetence which need treatment. By hand-held Doppler, incompetence of the saphenofemoral junction and of the junction between the short saphenous vein and the popliteal vein can be quickly demonstrated in outpatients. It is therefore good practice to have a pocket Doppler available when seeing patients with varicose veins.

DIFFERENTIAL DIAGNOSIS

Lipodermatosclerosis, hyperpigmentation, induration and venous ulceration are more often associated with chronic deep venous insufficiency and secondary varicosity than with simple varicose veins. A thrill or bruit may indicate the presence of an arteriovenous fistula but may be absent if the arteriovenous communication is small.

Venous dilatation which has appeared suddenly or become worse over a short period of time may be associated with extrinsic venous compression. The possibility should be particularly considered in the inguinal and retroperitoneal areas and evaluated with abdominal ultrasound and CT or MR scans.

Finally, venous engorgement in one limb without varicosity may be an indication of vascular compression of the venous system (e.g. compression by the right iliac artery crossing the left iliac vein; see p. 144).

Unilateral or bilateral swelling and oedema of the limbs may also be the result of a problem in the lymphatic system (see p. 146).

COMPLICATIONS

Acute
The main two are haemorrhage and thrombosis.

Haemorrhage

When the skin, especially in the perimalleolar area, becomes atrophic the varices become very superficial and are susceptible to even minor trauma. Rupture of the vein wall in such circumstances may cause exsanguinating bleeding because, if the patient remains standing, there is effectively a continuous uninterrupted column of blood from the right atrium to the ankle and blood flows freely retrograde through the incompetent venous system. It is essential that the limb is elevated and the site of bleeding compressed.

Thrombosis

A sudden incompressibility of dilated veins, usually associated with local pain and tenderness, is a sign that a varicose vein has thrombosed. The matter is considered in Chapter 9.

Chronic   Chronic complications of varicose veins are the consequence of long-standing venous hypertension and the accumulation of liquid in the interstitial space. Skin induration and hyperpigmentation (from the accumulation of haemosiderin which is released from extravasated red cells) finally leads to ulceration. Dermatitis, eczema and skin irritation are often associated with itching and scratch lesions may be seen. The affected skin is also susceptible to cellulitis and local infection.

TREATMENT   **General**

The aims are to:

- prevent continued high venous pressure in the superficial tissues with its effects on the microcirculation and nutrition (p. 126);
- relieve symptoms;
- improve the appearance of the leg.

Most patients (particularly young women) ask for treatment mainly for cosmetic reasons more than for symptoms and this should be taken into consideration. The type of therapy to be used is determined by the severity of the venous problem found. Some 30% of patients with simple varicosities do not require any therapy. Follow-up to establish if the changes found are progressive and to give advice are all that is needed.

Methods available   Three different modalities of treatment are commonly used: *non-operative management (drugs and physical measures), surgery and sclerotherapy*. The following rules must always be considered:

- Venous valvular insufficiency, of which varicose veins are a demonstration, is a chronic problem present throughout life. Therefore it is not possible in most patients to treat the problem with a single intervention. Rather, there should be repeated, planned therapy.
- It is more realistic to consider that the progression of venous insufficiency can be *controlled* rather than definitively treated either by non-operative management or by surgery and/or compression sclerotherapy.
- The three approaches must be well understood and logically applied in the different phases of the disorder and the life of the patient.
- Treatment must always be based on a careful understanding of the problem which is in turn the outcome of analysing the relative contributions of valvular incompetence and obstruction.

◆ Non-invasive investigation is the basis upon which correct treatment should be planned.

◆ Experience in all therapeutic approaches is essential so as to offer the optimum treatment which often requires sequential application of all three modalities.

◆ Treatment must always be planned, taking into consideration the fact that, with rare exceptions, the problem is not a dangerous one. Therefore, complications of therapy and unsatisfactory outcomes should be kept to a minimum.

Physical measures

Physical measures aim to reduce interstitial oedema, improve venous return and decrease the average venous pressure by encouraging the flow of blood from the varicose superficial system to the deep veins. Walking and regular physical exercise are useful while prolonged standing and sitting should be avoided. Elevating the leg whenever possible keeps venous pressure low and elastic stockings compress the superficial veins. Reflux through incompetent perforators is also reduced by effective compression. Below-knee stockings are very effective because the highest venous pressure and the most important varicosities form below the knee. By contrast, stockings are not very useful in compressing varicosities and perforators in the thigh. Elastic stockings are very helpful in controlling and preventing oedema and also improve the ability of the calf muscle pump to eject blood proximally. Elastic bandages can be used for compression in more severe cases and must be carefully applied by specialized staff so that they do not act as a tourniquet.

All the above measures are effective in most patients with simple varicose veins. Relief of symptoms and signs (particularly oedema) is generally rapidly obtained. Even in patients with more severe chronic venous hypertension, physical measures are not only palliative but may also constitute a very effective form of treatment when surgery or sclerotherapy are either not indicated or possible, or when patients refuse more aggressive forms of treatment.

Surgical treatment

Surgical treatment is indicated in the following circumstances:

◆ important symptoms and signs;

◆ very large varicosities which may thrombose to cause superficial thrombophlebitis;

◆ complications or a high risk of complications, e.g. a history of superficial thrombophlebitis or of haemorrhage from a ruptured varix;

◆ the presence of skin pigmentation, lipodermatosclerosis and/or ulceration;

◆ cosmesis.

Surgery for varicose veins aims to remove or ligate all (or the most important) varices and sites of incompetence between the deep and superficial systems. In secondary varicosities associated with deep venous valvular incompetence, the surgical control of the incompetent superficial veins must always be accompanied by some form of support for the limb and whenever possible by correction of the deep venous problem.

Stripping of the varicose veins is a debatable but very widely used procedure. It can be argued that to refrain from this procedure preserves a long saphenous vein which can be used in the future for a graft (peripheral vascular or coronary); however, a varicose great saphenous is very seldom useful for this purpose so there is little point in preserving it. It is therefore correct to use stripping when the whole long saphenous vein is varicose. Good results are obtained when stripping is performed correctly. With the patient standing, all incompetent varicosities and perforating veins must be identified and marked before surgery, a procedure that is made easier and more effective by the use of colour-duplex scanning to identify perforators. The operation (performed under general or regional anaesthesia) includes careful flush ligation of the saphenofemoral junction after division of all vessels that converge on the saphenofemoral opening (**Figure 5.1**). The trunk of the saphenous

Figure 5.1 High ligation (a) and section (b) of the saphenofemoral junction.

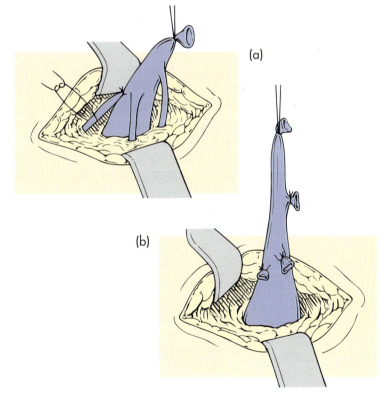

(a)

(b)

Figure 5.2 The long saphenous vein system (a) before and (b) during simple stripping. Most important venous trunks are left after stripping.

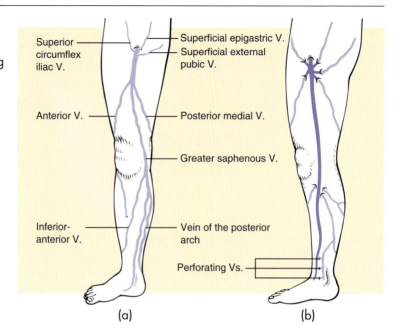

Superior circumflex iliac V.

Superficial epigastric V.
Superficial external pubic V.

Anterior V.

Posterior medial V.

Greater saphenous V.

Inferior-anterior V.

Vein of the posterior arch

Perforating Vs.

(a)   (b)

vein is removed after introducing an intraluminal stripper through a small incision at the ankle and passing this upwards to the divided vein in the groin.

As can be seen from **Figure 5.2**, many varicosities are not usually removed with stripping. The remaining varicose veins are removed or ligated through multiple small skin incisions. As an alternative and to avoid some skin incisions, these smaller remaining varicosities can be obliterated after a few weeks by sclerotherapy. However, some time should elapse before this is done because once the main high venous pressure segments have been ligated or removed most of the smaller low pressure tributaries tend to thrombose.

When other sites of deep to superficial incompetence are present, they are dealt with by ligation at the deep fascia or just deep to it—subfascial ligation.

These guidelines for the operation should be followed rigorously. Stripping applied blindly without making sure that incompetent communications are properly identified is likely to result in recurrence. However, limited stripping (associated with ligation of other incompetent venous sites) can be used (**Figure 5.3**). Limited stripping procedures are less traumatic, recovery is much quicker and the method is suitable for use as an outpatient procedure. Also, limited stripping preserves the segments of veins which are not varicose.

Incompetence of the lesser saphenous systems (**Figure 5.4**) is treated through incisions at the popliteal fold and behind the lateral malleolus and just below the popliteal fossa to strip the trunk,

Figure 5.3 Different types of stripping.

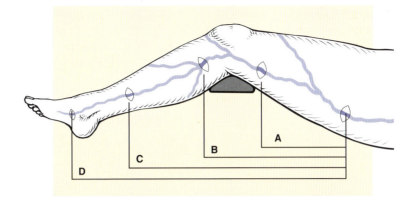

Figure 5.4 Massive varicosity at the popliteal fossa originating from an incompetent lesser saphenous vein.

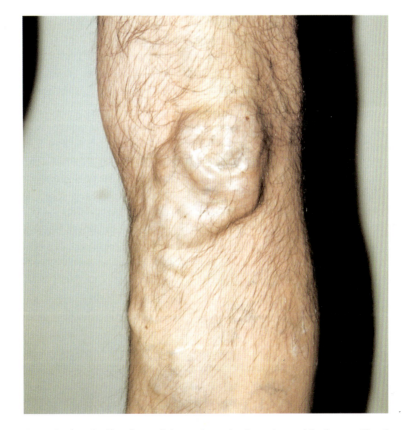

though simple ligation of the vein at its junction with the popliteal is often effective in reducing or abolishing varicosities. After a few weeks, sclerotherapy of residual veins is very effective in this area. As an alternative, stripping or multiple ligations of the incompetent veins (after ligating the saphenopopliteal junction) are satisfactory. Stripping of the lesser saphenous vein is more difficult than stripping of the long saphenous and damage to cutaneous nerves is more common.

Recurrences and the development of new varicosities are sometimes observed because variations of the anatomy in this area are numerous and the saphenopopliteal junction may be more proximal than expected. Ultrasound (colour-duplex scanning) and, in some circumstances such as surgery for recurrence, intraoperative venography may be very useful. These methods will correctly identify the branches present in the popliteal area, differentiating the popliteal vein and the gastrocnemius veins from the lesser saphenous and identifying its confluence into the deep system which is quite variable.

After surgery, elastic bandages or preferably graduated compression stockings (e.g. Siguaris or Kendall TED™) are generally used for a few days, depending on the extent of stripping and mainly to avoid postoperative haematomas. Thigh-length compression stockings or bandages are then worn for the following 2–4 weeks.

Physical measures such as elevation of the leg help to reduce postoperative pain and swelling. If the stripping has not been traumatic, most patients can walk after 4–6 hours and go home on the evening of the same day or early the next. The procedure, performed on an outpatient basis, may save costs and decrease bed occupancy in busy surgical wards. The limited period in bed decreases the possibility of postoperative deep venous thrombosis.

Other forms of treatment

Compression sclerotherapy obliterates veins by the action of a sclerosant in a collapsed channel. Permanent fibrosis takes place if the procedure is well performed. By contrast, if only thrombosis in the varix takes place, recanalization and recurrence are likely.

Method The varicose veins to be injected are marked with the patient standing. The patient is then placed supine and the sclerosing solution (0.5–1 ml of 3% sodium tetradecyl sulphate or polidocanol) is injected into the collapsed veins using a fine-gauge needle. The injected venous segment is isolated by digital pressure to keep the sclerosing solution in contact with the vein wall. A local compressive dressing of elastic adhesive (e.g. Tensoplast™) over a small cotton or paper swab is applied onto the injected area and leg compression with an elastic bandage or graduated compression stockings maintains the vein walls in contact until fibrosis has occurred. Compression prevents thrombophlebitis and fibrosis develops. After a period of between 2 and 4 weeks the elastic bandage may be removed. During the first session it is wise to inject only a minimal quantity of sclerosing agent so as to evaluate possible local and generalized reactions. Thereafter, several varices may be injected at each session.

Sclerotherapy is an outpatient procedure, is less expensive than surgical treatment and, if effective, the cosmetic result is the best of any method. In experienced hands, complications such as painful injections around the vein, skin pigmentation and ulceration are uncommon and easy to treat. Experience suggests that the short-term results of injection sclerotherapy are as good as those of surgery but long-term follow-up indicates a higher rate of recurrence. However, the two methods are not strictly comparable in that they have basically different indications. It is important to be able to use both methods according to the stage of venous disease and the needs of the individual patient. Ideally, compression sclerotherapy is more effective for small varices and dilated superficial veins, for below-knee perforators and for residual or recurrent veins after surgery. Sclerotherapy above the knee is often unsatisfactory because compression tends to be less effective. Surgical treatment gives better results for venous sites with severe incompetence such as the saphenofemoral junction, large perforators, or large varicose veins in direct communication with the main saphenous trunk.

Definition of minor and major incompetence

Any incompetent deep to superficial communications which modify the pattern of refilling time and AVP described in Chapter 4 are defined as sites of *major incompetence*. An example in the long saphenous system is shown in **Figure 5.5** where the AVP returns to its pre-exercise value in less than 14 seconds after exercise ceases. That this is limited to the saphenofemoral junction can be confirmed by compression with a thigh cuff which restores the refilling time and ambulatory pressure pattern to normal. Such findings indicate that ligation of the termination of the saphenous vein without stripping will be effective.

Figure 5.5 Ambulatory venous pressure measurements with and without a cuff excluding the superficial system.

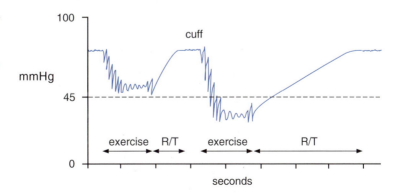

Figure 5.6 A large dilatation of an incompetent saphenofemoral junction.

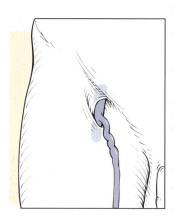

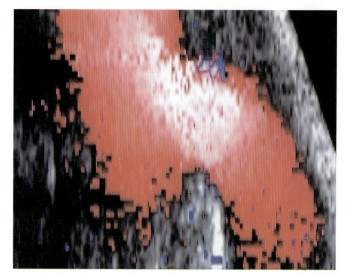

An alternative method of detection of major incompetence is to use colour-duplex with the patient standing to observe the quantity and duration of reflux on compression and its release. Considerable reflux lasting more than 3 seconds indicates a major incompetence (**Figure 5.6**). By contrast, communications that are not associated with modification of the AVP tracing and refilling time, or do so only in a minor way, are regarded as sites *of minor incompetence.* These can be very effectively treated with compression sclerotherapy with long-lasting results. Most residual varicosities after surgery are not associated with any abnormal pattern of AVP and therefore are, in general, suitable for sclerotherapy.

As an alternative to sclerotherapy or formal surgery, minor sites of incompetence can be treated through a small skin incision (1–2 mm) along the vein and the use of small hooks to extract and remove the vessel (Muller and Georgiev method). Stitches are not used and the cosmetic result is excellent. The procedure is an outpatient one and is very effective for veins associated with a low level of venous hypertension (**Figure 5.7**).

Sclerotherapy during surgery

Sclerotherapy can also be used during surgery to obliterate venous segments either distal or proximal to the point of ligation of major trunks (**Figure 5.8**) or to deal with small, distal venous segments (**Figure 5.9**). This use of sclerotherapy is very effective as recanalization is impeded by the ligation. Because reflux proximal to the site of sclerosis is absent, the period of elastic compression of the venous trunk after ligation can be shorter (1–2 weeks). This combined method is not frequently used but does offer an atraumatic

Figure 5.7 Varicose veins of the lower leg treated with local phlebectomy.
(a) Before; (b) 2 weeks after treatment.
(c) The hooks used to pull out the veins through a small incision (H. Georgiev method).

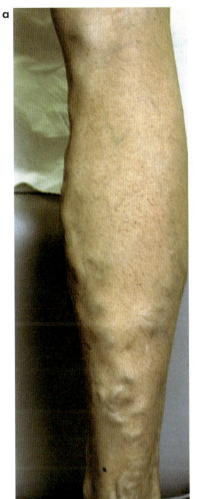
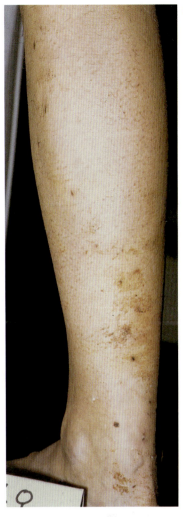
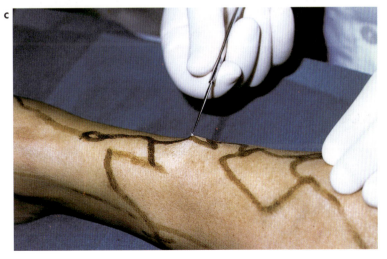

Figure 5.8 Infusion of sclerosing agent to obliterate a large collateral of the greater saphenous vein after ligation of the long saphenous vein.

Figure 5.9 Infusion into a smaller, below-knee branch during surgery after ligation.

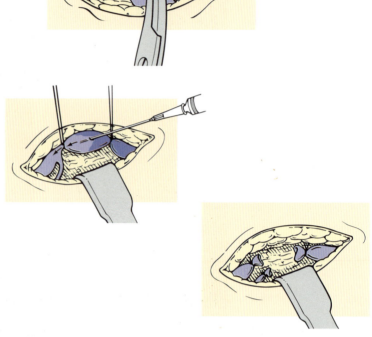

surgical procedure which combines ligation of the major sites of incompetence with simultaneous sclerotherapy of the residual veins.

Small varicosities and venous telangiectasis

Small 'capillary' veins (**Figure 5.10**) can be effectively treated with sclerotherapy. When the most important (usually central) vein of a cluster of dilatations is injected, all the veins in the area may disappear. Associated larger varicose veins are better treated first. Low concentration polidocanol (or other diluted sclerosing agent) is used and local compression maintained for a few days. A simple rule is as follows: the smallest venous dilatations—1 mm or less in diameter—are treated with 0.5–1% sclerosing agent and a week's compression; 1–2 mm receive 1–2% solution and 2 weeks of compression; for diameters in excess of 3 mm a 3% solution and 3 or more weeks of compression.

Red-pink very small vein dilatations are more difficult to treat than the 'blue' venular telangiectasias. Short- and long-term results after treatment tend to be much better with the latter.

Figure 5.10
(a) Infrared photograph of spider veins (venous telangiectasias). A small varicose vein is associated (arrows). These larger veins are usually sclerosed before treating the minor telangiectasias.

a

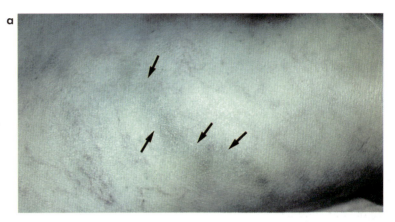

(b) The same area after treatment of the varicose veins and some telangiectasias.

b

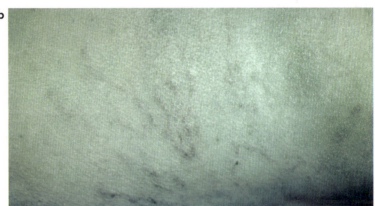

RESULTS AND PROGNOSIS

Because varicose veins are a continuing disorder, seldom treated with one single intervention, recurrence or the development of some new dilated or incompetent venous segments is relatively common. Even after well directed surgery, varicose veins recur in some 5–15% of patients. Therefore, it is good policy to see patients every year after an episode of treatment in order to identify developing varicosities and treat them (usually with sclerotherapy) before they become enlarged and cause a new cosmetic or clinical problem. A common cause of important recurrence is failure to ligate all tributaries of the greater saphenous system at the saphenofemoral junction. Failure to ligate other major incompetent perforators may also cause severe recurrence. Finally, recurrence may be the consequence of previously unrecognized deep venous hypertension which requires evaluation and possibly control or correction.

Drug treatment in varicose veins

This subject (and the general use of drugs in venous insufficiency) is discussed in Chapter 15. Venoactive drugs have a role before, after or in combination with compression, sclerotherapy and surgery. Drugs are not used to treat varicosity but to decrease the intensity of signs and symptoms due to the effects of chronic venous hypertension. Drugs effective on swelling (by reducing capillary filtration) are useful to control the development of oedema in many patients with varicose veins. There is also evidence that some drugs may be effective in improving venous wall tone but long-term clinical studies evaluating this parameter are not available. Effects of venoactive drugs on the microcirculation and on blood viscosity are useful both to relieve signs and symptoms, and to slow down the progression of chronic venous hypertension. Different drugs are available in different countries and the appropriate pharmaceutical database or guide should be consulted.

COMMENT   The debate between advocates of traditional surgery (such as stripping), of outpatient-based surgical techniques or of sclerotherapy is more or less irrelevant because, in a good unit offering a complete phlebological service, all methods of investigation and treatment should be equally and effectively made available to satisfy all clinical needs and the requirements of the patient. Also, it is important to remember that one single method does not cover all possible clinical situations and therefore it is useful to be skilled and experienced in all forms of treatment.

BIBLIOGRAPHY

Beaglehole R. Epidemiology of varicose veins. *World J Surg* 1986; **10**: 898.

Belcaro G, Laurora G, Cesarone MR, De Sanctis T, Incandela L. *Clinica Venosa*. Turin: Ediz. Minerva Medica, 1993.

Goren G, Yellin AE. Invaginated axial stripping and stab avulsion (hook) phlebectomy: a definitive outpatient procedure for primary varicose veins. *Ambulat Surg* 1993; **4**: 1.

Keith LM, Smead WL. Saphenous vein stripping and its complications. *Surg Clin North Am* 1983; **63**: 1303.

Plate G *et al*. Physiologic and therapeutic aspects in congenital vein valve aplasia of the lower limb. *Ann Surg* 1983; **198**: 229.

Sladen JG. Compression sclerotherapy: preparation, technique, complications and results. *Am J Surg* 1983; **146**: 228.

Thomas ML, Phillips GW. Recurrent groin varicose veins: an assessment by descending phlebography. *Br J Radiol* 1988; **61**: 294.

Tremblay J, Lewis EW, Allen PT. Selecting a treatment for primary varicose veins. *Can Med Assoc J* 1985; **133**: 20.

Wilkinson Jr GE, MacLaren IF. Long term review of procedures for venous perforator insufficiency. *Surg Gynecol Obstet* 1986; **163**: 11.

Williams RA, Wilson SE. Sclerosant treatment of varicose veins and deep vein thrombosis. *Arch Surg* 1984; **119**: 1283.

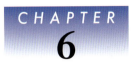
Deep venous thrombosis

**GENERAL
CONSIDERATIONS**

In the United States of America some 600 000 patients are treated each year in hospital for deep venous thrombosis. This and its sequel, pulmonary embolism, are common and sometimes fatal complications of major surgical procedures, particularly those followed by immobilization.

The three major factors considered to be the most important initiators of venous thrombosis were defined as long ago as 1856 by Virchow (**Table 6.1**):

Table 6.1 Situations and clinical problems that increase the risk of venous thrombosis

Vein wall alterations
    History of thrombosis
    Inflammation/infection around veins
    Venous trauma (cannulation or surgical)
    Varicose veins
Stasis
    All conditions associated with hypomobility
    Impairment in the mobility of limbs
    Congestive heart failure
    Extrinsic compression of veins by masses (tumours, abscesses, lymph nodes)
    Decreased arterial flow as in shock
Hypercoagulability
    Antithrombin III, protein S and protein C deficiency
    Surgery, trauma, injury
    Childbirth
    Hyperviscosity as in polycythaemia
    Neoplastic diseases
    Use of some contraceptives

♦ vein wall abnormalities—inflammation and trauma;
♦ blood flow alterations—reduction or turbulence;
♦ alterations in the properties of the blood—hypercoagulability, increased concentration of red cells, changes in viscosity.

The chain of events which produces venous thrombosis is summarized in **Figure 6.1**.

Venous thrombi are composed mainly of erythrocytes in a fibrin mesh with few platelets and are therefore known as *red thrombi*. By contrast, arterial thrombi are made up of platelet aggregates trapped in fibrin strands with only a few red cells (*white thrombi*). This indicates different mechanisms of their formation. The precise cause of a venous thrombosis is often difficult to determine. Thrombi may develop even in what appears to be a normal vein with a normal endothelium. Formation usually begins in the venous sinuses of the muscles of the legs and in the valve cusps (**Figure 6.2**) where venous flow is slow or the blood may even be temporarily static. In such areas an accumulation of activated clotting factors may occur. Platelets are important in the early phase of thrombus formation in that their aggregation triggers the coagulation process. As a platelet aggregate grows, it creates turbulent flow, so augmenting aggregation, which results in the release of

Figure 6.1 Factors involved in the haemostatic process.

Figure 6.2 Initial formation of a venous thrombus at valvular cusp.

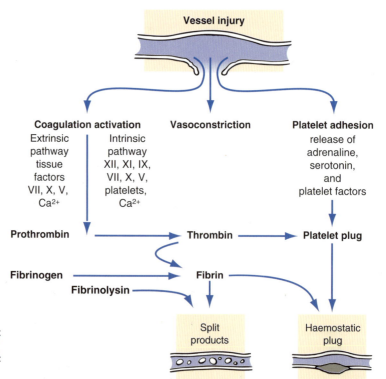

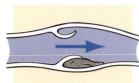

procoagulants and vasoconstrictor factors. The venous lumen is narrowed and blood flow is further reduced, so leading to a vicious circle of raised local coagulability and further accretion to the thrombus.

CLINICAL FEATURES The most important clinical matter when deep vein thrombosis is suspected is to establish clearly and as soon as possible that there definitely is a thrombus and whether in consequence management is required both to prevent pulmonary embolus and to treat the local problem.

The clinical features of thrombosis are variable. Symptoms are often absent. Most patients complain of pain and discomfort—made worse by exercise—in the involved calf or thigh. They may feel ill, with anxiety and fever.

The localization of the thrombus determines the most important physical findings. In the lower limbs, three main types of venous thrombosis, with different clinical pictures and development, can be identified (**Figure 6.3**):

◆ *localized calf thrombosis* may be confined to the sinuses of the soleal muscle and the posterior tibial and peroneal veins (**Figure**

Figure 6.3 Common patterns of venous thrombosis associated with different signs and symptoms.

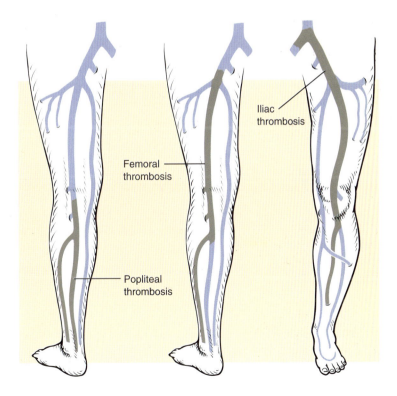

Iliac thrombosis

Femoral thrombosis

Popliteal thrombosis

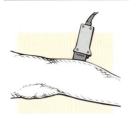

Figure 6.4 Initial calf thrombus (indicated by incompressibility of the soleal vein).

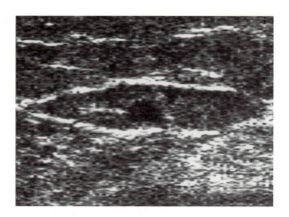

6.4). Calf tenderness may be present and distal swelling is slight or absent because obstruction of the main venous drainage of the limb has not yet occurred.

◆ *Femoral vein thrombosis* is often associated with calf thrombosis. There is pain and tenderness in the distal thigh and popliteal region. Swelling is more prominent than with calf vein thrombosis alone and can extend to the level of the knee.

◆ *Iliofemoral venous thrombosis* produces the most severe manifestations, often with massive swelling and tenderness of the entire lower extremity.

Phlegmasia cerulea dolens is an especially severe form of iliofemoral thrombosis that produces such marked obstruction to venous outflow that cyanosis develops. It can progress to *venous gangrene* in which there is loss of superficial tissue though rarely of the whole limb. *Phlegmasia alba dolens* is another variant characterized by arterial spasm or compression because of massive oedema: the leg is pale and cool with diminished or absent pulses. Irreversible ischaemia may take place.

Especially in early thrombosis, the clinical signs are often unreliable. Occasionally, tenderness to palpation along any of the involved veins may be observed. With thrombosis in the calf, active dorsiflexion of the foot often produces calf pain (Homans' sign); similarly, tenderness of the calf when the muscles are compressed against the tibia may be a first clue to the presence of thrombosis. However, both are unreliable indicators.

Differences in the circumference of the affected extremity compared to the unaffected one are often detectable by measurement. This is possibly the most reliable diagnostic sign.

As collateral venous flow develops, the superficial veins are sometimes visibly dilated and, if the inflammatory component is significant, there may be increased local warmth and erythema.

DIAGNOSTIC TESTS   Clinical diagnosis is not reliable: at an early stage most patients have no symptoms and the clinical signs are slight and misleading. An objective diagnostic test should be used to establish the presence of thrombosis and the need for treatment.

Continuous wave ultrasound   A pocket Doppler can identify reduced or obstructed flow in major veins and is a simple and quick way to search for large occlusive thrombi. In expert hands it is accurate 80–85% of the time, is inexpensive and can be repeated frequently. In obstruction of the iliac, femoral or popliteal veins the normal respiratory fluctuations in venous flow are abolished and the augmented flow in response to compression of distal muscles such as those in the calf is absent. However, thrombosis that does not produce obstruction cannot be detected with Doppler. Confusing results may occur when a thrombus partially obstructs the vein or when extensive collateral venous flow is present (**Figure 6.5**). Continuous-wave Doppler also cannot be used accurately as a screening or diagnostic method for localized calf vein thrombosis and generally for any thrombosis not associated with some degree of obstruction.

B-mode ultrasound   This can reveal the incompressibility of veins under compression with the probe, the presence of a visible thrombus (echogenicity), and the lack of venous distension with a Valsalva manoeuvre (indicating iliac or femoral thrombosis). All are reliable criteria of

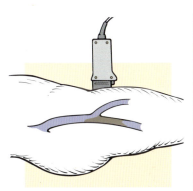

Figure 6.5 Common femoral vein occluded by a thrombus. The long saphenous vein (in blue) is patent.

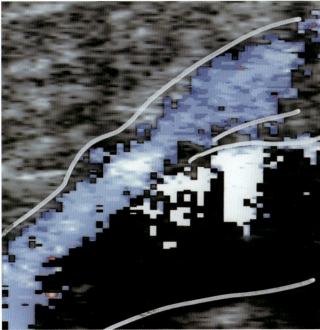

thrombosis. The B-mode demonstration of femoral or popliteal vein thrombosis indicates the need for anticoagulation (see pp. 80–82). Localized iliac vein thrombosis may not be detected by B-mode imaging alone but should be correctly diagnosed by Doppler flow evaluation.

Duplex and colour-duplex ultrasound

Duplex and colour-duplex ultrasound combine B-mode with Doppler flow imaging. Colour-flow imaging also visualizes the direction of flow, turbulence and flow variations with compression and with respiration. Duplex and colour-duplex are very accurate in the detection of major axial vein thrombosis (sensitivity and specificity rates are 90–100%). Colour-duplex is faster and more accurate.

With colour-duplex, after scanning the femoral veins in the supine position and the popliteal vein on standing (weight on the opposite limb—though there are circumstances in which this is not possible), scanning all the remaining main superficial and deep veins of both legs in a sitting position (**Figure 6.6**) requires about 20 minutes. Then, using a 3.5 MHz probe, the iliac veins and the inferior vena cava are scanned with the patient supine. In most patients it is possible easily to scan the intra-abdominal veins, so obtaining results that are comparable with phlebography. Particularly with colour-duplex, the flow around the thrombus on compression of the calf allows a very clear and rapid visualization of thrombosis, better demonstrating floating thrombi which may cause embolism (**Figures 6.7** and **6.8**).

Figure 6.6 Position to scan the most important deep veins. During the test the muscles must be relaxed.

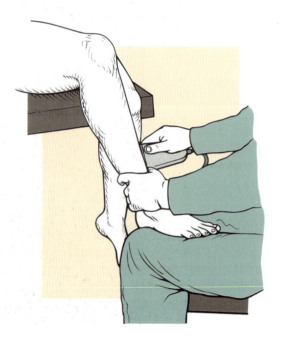

Figure 6.7
Thrombus in the
popliteal vein shown
by phlebography (a);
B-mode ultrasound (b);
and colour-duplex (c).
The blue colour in (c)
indicates the passage
of blood around the
thrombus during
manual compression
of the calf.

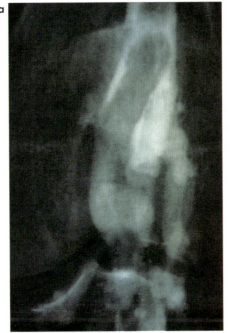 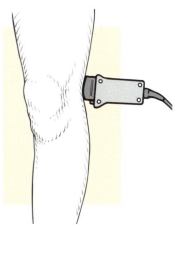

a

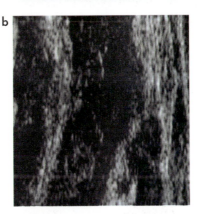 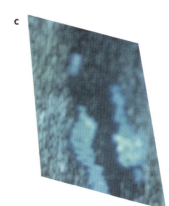

b c

Figure 6.8 A free-
floating thrombus in
the femoral vein. The
venous flow around the
edge of the thrombus
indicates no contact
between the thrombus
and the venous wall.

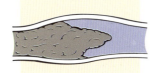 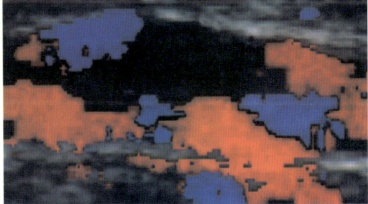

The demonstration of thrombosis in the upper limb or subclavian veins and those draining into the superior vena cava is relatively more difficult and less precise.

Ascending phlebography

There is no reason to ask for a phlebogram when the diagnosis has been established by non-invasive investigation in that the most important and frequent problem in such circumstances is to decide what type of treatment (i.e. anticoagulation) should be used. In that phlebography may have complications, it is inappropriate to undertake it unless there is a good and compelling reason (e.g. to modify treatment or to decide what type of surgical procedure is needed). Additional disadvantages are expense, the possibility that the procedure may cause thrombosis and inability to repeat the investigation at frequent intervals. Hence it is unsuitable as a screening method.

Whenever possible, the test is done with the patient standing and the weight on the other extremity. The contrast medium is injected into a vein on the dorsum of the foot. Calf, popliteal, femoral and iliac veins are visualized. Thrombosis is indicated by:

◆ constant filling defects;
◆ diversion of flow;
◆ abrupt termination of the contrast column;
◆ failure to fill either the entire deep system or segments of it.

The phlebographic appearance of a thrombus in the popliteal vein in comparison with images obtained with B-mode duplex and colour-duplex is shown in **Figure 6.7**. The sinuses and small veins of the calf muscles are difficult to visualize and the deep femoral vein is opacified in only 50% of patients. However, in that phlebography demonstrates over 90% of thrombi, it is considered the most accurate method of investigation. A negative venogram generally excludes the presence of thrombosis in the lower extremities.

Radionuclide venography

This is simpler and appears to be accurate and reliable in detecting major vein occlusion. Both contrast and radionuclide venography can generally be done, when circumstances permit, on an outpatient basis.

Plethysmography

The technique detects obstruction to outflow of blood from the leg by measuring the changes in the volume of venous flow. However, all plethysmographic methods may be negative in proximal thrombosis associated with good collateral circulation.

Air plethysmography (see Chapter 3) has recently been used for the non-invasive diagnosis of venous thrombosis and to quantify venous obstruction with good results.

Impedance plethysmography calculates the volume of blood in the limb by measuring changes in electrical resistance and can detect iliac, femoral and popliteal thrombosis which are the most important sources of pulmonary emboli. A positive result is correct in at least 90% of patients with major thrombi producing obstruction. However, impedance plethysmography is not accurate for the evaluation of calf thrombosis because it is insensitive to partial occlusion of a vein. Plethysmography has been replaced in many vascular centres by tests based on ultrasound. However, it is still widely used in the United States of America though its application in Europe is limited.

Radioactive fibrinogen (RF) test

Circulating fibrinogen becomes incorporated into growing thrombi. If fibrinogen is labelled with a radioactive material (^{125}I), thrombosis can be detected by external scanning over the veins. The test is both highly sensitive and specific and reveals even small, localized soleal, tibial and peroneal vein thrombosis. In consequence it has been used as the standard with which other investigations can be compared and it correlates well with venography. Its practical diagnostic application is, however, limited because between 12 and 24 hours are required between administration and completion. Moreover, it cannot detect a thrombus that is not incorporating fibrinogen. Finally, there is still some debate as to whether all radioactive fibrinogen accumulations should be regarded as thromboses and whether they constitute an indication for treatment.

Screening with RF indicates that deep venous thrombosis may occur in some 30–60% of general surgical and in 50% of orthopaedic or neurosurgical patients and often begins during surgery. Clinical features are present in only 5–10% of these subjects. About 90% of postoperative thrombi detected by the RF test are localized to the calf at diagnosis. Only 20% progress to the larger veins (popliteal or femoral) to produce clinical features and to become a potential source of emboli.

Blood tests

Blood tests have been developed to detect intravascular coagulation including measurement of *fibrinopeptide A, circulating fibrin monomer complexes* and *serum fibrin degradation products.* Measurement of the degradation product fragment E is a sensitive test but the method is complex and unsuitable for clinical work. All blood tests lack specificity.

Monoclonal antibody-labelled platelets and fibrin

These can be used to localize thrombi. The development of methods based on these substances may have applications not only in the limbs but also elsewhere in the body, for example, the brain.

Other tests   Deep venous thrombosis may be the consequence of an abdominal tumour compressing the iliac veins or the inferior vena cava. Causes of venous compression, such as intra-abdominal masses, should always be seriously considered, particularly in elderly patients. Abdominal ultrasound scans, MRI and CT scans are useful to demonstrate extrinsic compression and should be used to evaluate surgical conditions before initiating anticoagulant or fibrinolytic treatment.

DIFFERENTIAL
DIAGNOSIS   The clinical presentation of venous thrombosis is very variable and often signs and symptoms are mild or absent.

Compression by a synovial cyst (Baker's cyst) (**Figure 6.9**) on the popliteal vein may mimic a popliteal thrombosis as may acute synovial rupture and extravasation of synovial fluid into the calf muscles (*pseudothrombophlebitis syndrome*). These patients often have arthropathy of the knee with effusion and a popliteal mass may be palpable. Ultrasound and arthrography are useful to establish the diagnosis.

Contusion of a calf muscle, rupture of the tendon of the plantaris muscle and *haematomas* (**Figure 6.10**) can produce a swollen, painful calf and may be difficult to differentiate from deep venous occlusion. Acute onset of symptoms during exercise and ecchymo-

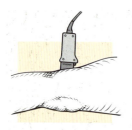

Figure 6.9 Ultrasound image of a Baker's cyst.

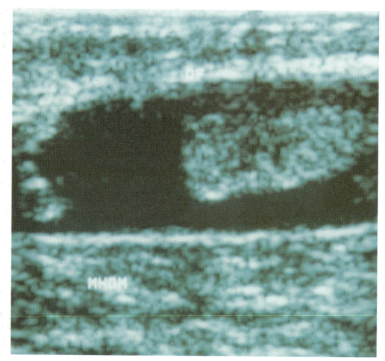

sis in the calf are suggestive of muscle injury. However, ultrasound to confirm that the popliteal vein is compressible and occasionally phlebography may be required.

Lymphatic or systemic conditions may cause swelling of a limb (Chapter 12). Bilateral swelling is sometimes seen in bilateral iliac or caval venous thrombosis but it is more usually of cardiac or renal origin. When *cellulitis* is present, swelling may be acute and associated with pain, inflammation and often a wound. Occasionally it is difficult to distinguish an *arterial occlusion* from a venous one. Usually arterial occlusion is associated with more pain and early loss of sensation. There is absence of swelling, the superficial veins are not distended and refill very slowly when emptied; by contrast, in venous thrombosis they are full and dilated. The pocket Doppler may be helpful in rapidly establishing the correct diagnosis.

Duplex and colour-duplex scanning are very effective in differentiating venous thrombosis from other vascular problems. It is only occasionally necessary to resort to venography. A great advantage of duplex and colour-duplex over venography is that the test may be easily repeated after 24–48 hours when there is doubt. Identification of a patent venous system by duplex/colour-duplex may avoid anticoagulation or hospital admission with great advantage for the patient and the costs of health care.

Figure 6.10 A calf haematoma.

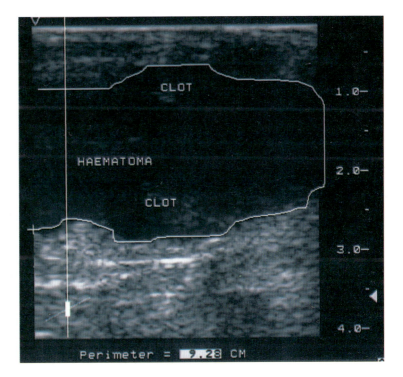

MANAGEMENT

General

The aims of treatment are to prevent the progression of thrombosis, the formation of additional or new thrombi, to prevent embolization and to avoid as far as possible damage to the valves of the deep veins. In relation to pulmonary embolus the risk of mortality appears to increase with the proximity of the thrombus to the heart. Ventilation/perfusion scans have demonstrated pulmonary embolization in about 30% of calf, about 50% of iliofemoral and in about 65% of inferior vena cava thromboses.

Physical measures

It takes some 7–8 days for experimental thrombi to become firmly adherent to vein walls and therefore it is common practice to advise bed rest for about a week after the onset of symptoms. The feet are elevated 10–20° above the level of the heart. This measure appears to reduce oedema and pain and the increased venous flow lessens the possibility of new thrombus formation. Elastic compression of the limb is indicated because it decreases venous accumulation and increases the velocity of venous flow. Bed rest should be continued until swelling, pain and tenderness have been reduced. Ambulation with elastic compression (graduated compression stockings) is then permitted, avoiding standing and sitting with the legs dependent because any sustained increase in venous pressure aggravates oedema and discomfort. Elastic support and limitations on sitting and standing are generally advised for 3–6 months until recanalization and collateral veins develop.

Anticoagulant therapy

Unless there are specific contraindications, anticoagulants should be initiated as soon as possible in every thrombosis which may be potentially a cause of pulmonary embolism. The aims of anticoagulation are:

◆ to prevent the growth of the thrombus;
◆ to avoid the development of new thrombi;
◆ to prevent pulmonary embolization.

Anticoagulation has the additional advantage that it hastens dissolution of the thrombus by allowing endogenous fibrinolysis to operate unopposed.

Standard heparin

Heparin therapy should be started as soon as the diagnosis of deep venous thrombosis has been confirmed. Heparin inhibits thrombus formation by neutralizing thrombin, by blocking the formation of thromboplastin and by inhibiting the release of coagulation factors from platelets. It is of proven benefit in the treatment of deep venous thrombosis and the prevention of pulmonary embolism. It is not absorbed from the gastrointestinal tract, therefore must be given either intravenously or subcutaneously. The former is clearly more effective and its effects on clotting are immediate. Intramuscular injections of heparin should be avoided as they may cause local haemorrhage at the injection site. An initial loading dose of 100 units/kg body weight should be given intravenously and subsequent doses determined by laboratory tests which may include the whole blood clotting time, the activated partial thromboplastin time (APTT) or activated clotting time (ACT). Progression of the thrombus and the occurrence of pulmonary embolism are minimized by administering sufficient heparin to maintain the APTT at least at 1.5 times the control value. The amount of heparin required may vary from day to day; therefore, the state of anticoagulation should be monitored at least daily. Most patients initially require 1000–2000 units per hour to achieve adequate anticoagulation.

A less satisfactory alternative to continuous intravenous heparin is bolus therapy. The drug should be given every 4 or 6 hours and the test of coagulation performed 1 hour before the next scheduled dose. For acute deep vein thrombosis, heparin is usually administered for 7–10 days, the time required for thrombi to become firmly adherent to the vein walls. However, a 5-day course has been shown, by prospective randomized studies, to be as effective. If, after 5–10 days, symptoms and signs such as pain and tenderness are still present, or repeated ultrasound tests indicate growth or extension of the thrombus, heparin should be continued.

If pulmonary embolism has occurred, larger doses of heparin are used and treatment is continued for up to 3 weeks. Even under effective heparin treatment the incidence of pulmonary embolism may reach 5%.

Complications of heparin therapy

Bleeding is the most important complication but is less common if the heparin is given by continuous intravenous infusion. It occurs in 5–10% of patients, particularly in those who have undergone surgery or who have a lesion in the gastrointestinal or genitourinary tract. The most usual cause, however, is that too much heparin has been administered. Bleeding may be an important sign of an undiagnosed neoplastic or ulcerated lesion. Protamine sulphate, a heparin inhibitor, is given when bleeding is significant.

Antiplatelet drugs which diminish platelet aggregation may, in heparinized patients, interfere with primary haemostasis and coagulation. Platelet counts should be obtained before and during heparin therapy because thrombocytopenia—caused by a heparin-induced antiplatelet antibody which leads to platelet aggregation—

may occur within hours or days after heparin is started. It may be persistent and severe and is sometimes associated with severe bleeding, recurrent thrombosis or pulmonary embolism.

Low-molecular-weight heparins

Low-molecular-weight heparins are associated with fewer bleeding complications.

Oral anticoagulants

The coumarin derivatives block synthesis in the liver of at least four vitamin K-dependent clotting factors: prothrombin and factors VII, IX and X. The anticoagulant effects are delayed until these factors have been cleared from the blood and therefore the onset of action of oral anticoagulants is slow. The treatment reduces the prothrombin time and is used for long-term prophylaxis or continued treatment after discontinuing heparin. Oral anticoagulants inhibit the synthesis of the anticoagulant protein C and its cofactor S. Protein C has a very short half-life and in consequence there is a period of relative hypercoagulability during the first days of treatment with oral anticoagulant. Therefore bishydroxycoumarin (warfarin), the most commonly used drug, should be started during the first or second day of heparin treatment and the latter discontinued only after the prothrombin time has been at therapeutic levels for a few days. The therapeutic range for oral anticoagulants is controversial. The commonly recommended dose is one which increases the prothrombin time to 2–2.5 times the normal value but this is probably excessive. An equal antithrombotic effect can be achieved with a prothrombin time of 1.35–1.6. Many laboratories report the *International Normalized Ratio (INR)* as well as the prothrombin time. The INR takes into consideration variations in reactivity of reagents used to determine prothrombin time and has been suggested by British and European haematologists as the appropriate reference standard. However, it is not commonly accepted by many North American institutions or quoted in their medical journals or books. If the INR is used, the recommended level for therapy of deep venous thrombosis is 2–3.

Duration of anticoagulant therapy

After a deep venous thrombosis, oral anticoagulation should be continued for at least 3 months because this is the time required for the development of venous collaterals and is also the period during which most recurrences occur. After pulmonary embolism, 6 months of anticoagulation is indicated.

Complications of oral anticoagulant therapy

Bleeding occurs in 5–10% of patients. Excessive prolongation of the prothrombin time is urgently treated with vitamin K but adjusting the dose of anticoagulant may be enough if bleeding is mild. Consideration should be given to altering the regimen to self-administered, low-dose heparin therapy as an alternative to oral anticoagulants in the long-term management of thromboembolic disorders because this appears to be associated with fewer bleeding complications. Apart from bleeding, the major problem is drug interaction. There are many commonly used agents that interact with oral anticoagulants usually (but not always) to potentiate their activity. Amongst these are H_2 receptor blockers, non-steroidal anti-inflammatory agents, some antibiotics and barbiturates. A careful drug history must be taken and the current intake known.

Recurrent thromboembolism occurs in less than 2% of patients treated effectively.

Fibrinolytic activators   Fibrinolytic activators (streptokinase, urokinase) produce lysis of fresh thrombi. Rapid clearance of any occluded veins can result and competence and function of venous valves may be better preserved than with heparin treatment. Therefore, fibrinolytic therapy may be an effective method of preventing the post-thrombotic syndrome. Prospective studies suggest that normal venous function is preserved in about 40% of patients after fibrinolytic therapy. However, fibrinolysis has no advantage over heparin when venous thrombosis had been present for more than 72 hours nor is it any more effective in preventing recurrence. Particularly in surgical patients, bleeding complications are more common than with conventional anticoagulation.

Streptokinase is antigenic and should only be used after a test dose has been administered. An alternative is *tissue plasminogen activator (tPA)* made by recombinant DNA techniques and which is not only more specific for the site of thrombosis but also possibly faster in its action.

The use of all types of fibrinolytic therapy is expensive. Studies are at present in progress on catheter-directed fibrinolysis for an identified segment of thrombosis in a large vein.

Ancrod (Arvin)   This is a proteinase derived from the venom of the pit viper which accelerates the conversion of factor X into Xa and thus leads to the conversion of fibrinogen into fibrin and its degradation products. Depletion of circulating fibrinogen results in a hypocoagulable state—blood is essentially *defibrinated*. Ancrod has been used successfully in the management of deep venous thrombosis but it does not appear to be superior to heparin. Currently its use is on a 'named patient' basis and is restricted to clinical trials.

Bleeding complications should be treated with Arvin Antidote (which may cause anaphylaxis), freeze-dried fibrinogen or, if this is not available, fresh plasma.

COMPLICATIONS OF DEEP VEIN THROMBOSIS

The most important *acute* complications are pulmonary embolism and severe outflow obstruction leading to venous gangrene. The only *chronic* complication is chronic venous insufficiency (post-phlebitic syndrome) which may lead to secondary varicosity (see varicose veins, Chapter 5) and ulceration (Chapter 11).

Surgical treatment

The majority of patients are managed by anticoagulation which is effective in the relief of local symptoms and the prevention of pulmonary embolism. However, lysis of the thrombus depends on the endogenous thrombolytic system and requires weeks or months and leads to recanalization with destruction of the venous valves present in the affected segment. Therefore, anticoagulation is of little value in preventing the post-thrombotic syndrome that will inevitably follow the loss of valve function. As already described, thrombolytic therapy seems to be the logical way to solve this problem but more research is needed to prove its efficacy.

In acute iliofemoral thrombosis there is a revival of interest in *surgical thrombectomy* (Eklof) combined with a temporary arteriovenous fistula. The objectives are to prevent fatal pulmonary embolism, further swelling of the leg with development of an acute compartment syndrome which may lead to phlegmasia cerulea dolens and venous gangrene, and to prevent post-thrombotic syndrome. The current indications are if the history of swelling of the thigh indicates that iliac obstruction is less than 7 days in duration and the activity expectancy of the patient is more than 10 years.

Several studies indicate no mortality from peroperative pulmonary embolism and no difference in non-fatal pulmonary embolism compared with control groups treated only by anticoagulation.

Surgery has an immediate positive effect on swelling of the leg and it is certainly indicated if phlegmasia cerulea dolens has already developed. Thrombectomy has shown a significant improvement of iliac vein patency and valvular function and should in consequence prevent the development of the post-thrombotic syndrome.

Venous interruption

The rationale is the prevention of recurrent and potentially fatal pulmonary embolism by trapping a detached clot in the peripheral venous segments. In patients with a single pulmonary embolus treated with effective anticoagulation, fatal pulmonary embolism is rare (1–2%). Venous interruption is indicated for the patient who fails to respond to anticoagulants or who has specific contraindications to their use and in whom thrombectomy is regarded as inappropriate.

Figure 6.11 Secondary prevention of pulmonary embolism with partial interruption of the vena cava to trap large emboli. The Moretz caval clip and the Miles Teflon clip (middle, lower) are among those most commonly used. They are usually placed just distally to the renal veins. The gonadal veins should be ligated. The Greenfield intracaval filter (right part of the figure) may be inserted transcutaneously.

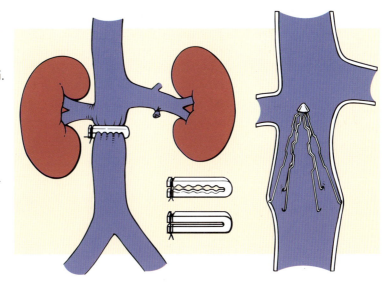

Ligation of the superficial femoral vein prevents embolization from distal muscular and deep veins and is rarely followed by chronic venous insufficiency. However, this procedure cannot prevent embolization from more proximal venous segments. In that most fatal pulmonary emboli arise from the iliac or pelvic veins, venous interruption in the extremities has been replaced by techniques that trap emboli distally (**Figure 6.11**). Ligation of the inferior vena cava (IVC) was first introduced by Homans in 1944 and since then numerous methods for interruption which are short of such a drastic intervention have been developed and applied. The advantages of preserving flow in the IVC and not producing a raised distal venous pressure stimulated the development of plication techniques using sutures or serrated clips placed surgically. The Adams–De Weese clips are still used. The alternative is transvenous placement of a filter which, to be effective, must arrest emboli large enough to produce haemodynamic effects if they were to reach the lungs, maintain IVC patency and remain in position. The early devices, such as the Hunter balloon and the Mobir–Udin umbrella, were either susceptible to proximal migration or produced an unacceptable morbidity from occlusion of the IVC. Currently, however, there are satisfactory devices of sufficiently small size to be safely introduced percutaneously.

The indications for insertion of a vena cava filter vary, being more liberal in the USA than in Europe. In patients with objective documentation of deep venous thrombosis or at least one pulmonary embolism there are the following currently accepted indications:

♦ problems with anticoagulation:
contraindication,
failure,
complications;
♦ prophylaxis in patients with deep venous thrombosis who would be at high risk of death if they were to sustain a pulmonary embolus;
♦ following pulmonary embolectomy.

Comparison of different filters is difficult because prospective randomized studies have not been performed and investigation of individual filters differs in indications for placement, follow-up and the population from which the patients are drawn. The Greenfield stainless steel filter was introduced in 1972 and the information on long-term follow-up for this device is the current standard for implantable vena caval devices. It has a greater than 90% efficiency in the prevention of further pulmonary embolism after an initial episode and a patency rate of the same order.

Other filters currently available are the Nitinol filter (1977; **Figure 6.12**), the Gunther filter (1983), the 'birds nest' filter (1984), the Venatech filter (1986) and the titanium Greenfield filter (1989). None of these has so far been proven superior and the filter most likely to prevent recurrent pulmonary embolism and the least likely to cause caval thrombosis has yet to be defined.

Figure 6.12 The Nitinol caval filter.

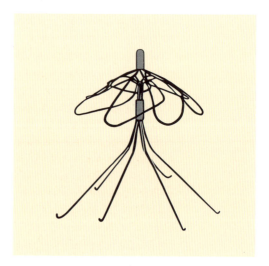

BIBLIOGRAPHY

Barnes RW *et al.* Peri-operative asymptomatic venous thrombosis: role of duplex scanning versus venography. *J Vasc Surg* 1989; **9:** 251.

Bergqvist D, Comerota A, Nicolaides AN, Scurr J. *Prevention of Venous Thromboembolism.* European Workshop and Consensus Statement. London: Med-Orion, 1994.

Browse NL. Prevention of postoperative deep vein thrombosis. *Br J Surg* 1988; **75:** 835.

Colditz GA, Tuden RL, Oster G. Rates of venous thrombosis after general surgery: combined results of randomised clinical trials. *Lancet* 1986; **2:** 143.

Cole CW, Bormanis J. Ancrod: a practical alternative to heparin. *J Vasc Surg* 1988; **8:** 59.

Collins R *et al.* Reduction in fatal pulmonary embolism and venous thrombosis by peri-operative administration of subcutaneous heparin. *N Engl J Med* 1988; **318:** 1162.

Coon WW. Venous thromboembolism: prevalence, risk factors, and prevention. *Clin Chest Med* 1984; **5:** 391.

Duckert F. Thrombolytic therapy. *Semin Thromb Hemost* 1984; **10:** 87.

Eklof B. The value of thrombectomy. In: Bergqvist D, Comerota A, Nicolaides AN, Scurr J, cds. *Prevention of Venous Thromboembolism.* European Workshop and Consensus Statement. London: Med-Orion, 1994; 357.

Engesser L *et al.* Hereditary protein S deficiency: clinical manifestations. *Ann Intern Med* 1987; **106:** 677.

Ginsberg JS, Hirsh J. Anticoagulants during pregnancy. *Ann Rev Med* 1989; **40:** 79.

Goldhaber SZ *et al.* Pooled analyses of randomized trials of streptokinase and heparin in phlebographically documented acute deep venous thrombosis. *Am J Med* 1984; **76:** 393.

Graor R. Fibrinolytic therapy for deep vein thrombosis and pulmonary embolism. *Cardiovasc Intervent Radiol* 1988; **11:** 533.

Greenfield LJ. Current indications for and results of Greenfield filter placement. *J Vasc Surg* 1984; **1:** 502.

Greenfield LJ, Alexander EL. Current status of surgical therapy for deep vein thrombosis. *Am J Surg* 1985; **150:** 64.

Greenfield LJ *et al.* Preliminary clinical experiences with the titanium Greenfield filter. *Arch Surg* 1989; **124:** 657.

Harris WH *et al.* Prophylaxis of deep vein thrombosis after total hip replacement: dextran and external pneumatic compression compared with 1.2 or 0.3 g aspirin daily. *J Bone Joint Surg* 1985; **67:** 57.

Hirsh J. New approach for deep vein thrombosis occurring after surgery. *JAMA* 1984; **251:** 2895.

Hull RD *et al.* A cost-effectiveness analysis of alternative approaches for long term treatment of proximal venous thrombosis. *JAMA* 1984; **25:** 235.

Hull RD *et al.* Continuous intravenous heparin compared with intermittent subcutaneous heparin in the initial treatment of proximal vein thrombosis. *N Engl J Med* 1986; **315:** 1109.

Inada K *et al.* Effects of intermittent pneumatic leg compression for prevention of postoperative deep venous thrombosis with special reference to fibrinolytic activity. *Am J Surg* 1988; **155:** 602.

Killewich LA *et al.* Diagnosis of deep venous thrombosis; a prospective study comparing duplex scanning to contrast venography. *Circulation* 1989; **79:** 810.

Killewich LA *et al.* Spontaneous lysis of deep venous thrombi. Rate of outcome. *J Vasc Surg* 1989; **9:** 89.

Lensing AWA *et al.* Detection of deep vein thrombosis by real time B-mode ultrasound. *N Engl J Med* 1989; **320:** 342.

Orsini RA, Jarrell BE. Suprarenal placement of vena cava filters: indications, techniques and results. *J Vasc Surg* 1984; **1:** 124.

Plate G *et al.* Thrombectomy with temporary arteriovenous fistula. The treatment of choice in acute iliofemoral venous thrombosis. *J Vasc Surg* 1984; **1:** 867.

Rohrer MJ *et al.* Extended indications for placement of an inferior vena cava filter. *J Vasc Surg* 1989; **10:** 44.

Rollins DL *et al.* Origin of deep vein thrombi in an ambulatory population. *Am J Surg* 1988; **156:** 122.

Siderow J. Streptokinase vs heparin for deep vein thombosis. Can lytic therapy be justified? *Arch Intern Med* 1989; **149:** 1841.

Wakentin TE *et al.* Percutaneous placement of the Greenfield vena cava filter. *Mayo Clin Proc* 1988; **63:** 343.

White RH *et al.* Diagnosis of deep vein thrombosis using duplex ultrasound. *Ann Intern Med* 1989; **111:** 2979.

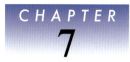

CHAPTER 7

Pulmonary thromboembolism

GENERAL CONSIDERATIONS

It is estimated that fatal pulmonary embolism (PE) occurs every year in more than 600 000 patients in the USA where it is the third most frequent cause of death and is responsible for at least 5% of postoperative deaths of which a quarter to a half occur in patients with a good prognosis. Non-fatal attacks are 3 – 5 times more frequent than fatal ones. Pulmonary thromboembolism is therefore relatively common and can occur in almost any clinical setting. However, it is rare in healthy young patients while elderly, immobilized, sick, or traumatized patients have the highest incidence.

Deep venous thrombosis of the legs, demonstrated only in 30 – 40% of patients with PE, is the most common cause of embolization. Immobilization in bed and decreased ambulant mobility and exercise may double the incidence of PE. A higher risk is also present during pregnancy and in the puerperium. Heart disease of all kinds, cardiac failure, surgical procedures, the use of oral contraceptives and having blood group A are other factors which increase the risk of PE.

The iliac and femoral veins are the source of most pulmonary emboli but clots can also originate in other systemic veins, such as in an axillary–subclavian venous thrombosis. Thrombosis confined to smaller veins (e.g. the calf) rarely cause severe PE. It is only thrombi produced in veins the size of the iliac and femoral that are large enough to cause emboli with major clinical sequelae.

Much rarer causes of PE are *tumour embolization of the lungs* usually from a renal cell carcinoma and *cardiac tumours* such as myxomas in the right atrium or ventricle. In most patients PE involves lobar arteries in each lung.

Pulmonary embolism and infarction are different clinical entities in that less than 10% of pulmonary emboli produce infarction that is an ischaemic area of lung. A true pulmonary infarct is seldom produced in a normal lung and even ligation of the pulmonary artery does not lead to infarction. Infarcts are usually peripheral and most often in the lower lobes. They occur when occlusion of a pulmonary artery takes place in the presence of a severe clinical condition affecting the lung (e.g. chronic lung disease, infection or congestive heart failure). Because occlusion of a pulmonary artery affects respiration, the global pulmonary circulation, the heart and the bronchial circulation, several different mechanisms are involved in the response to a PE.

Changes which involve pulmonary reflexes—such as vasoconstriction with consequent pulmonary hypertension and changes in respiratory rate—are probably secondary to microembolization. Vasoactive amines and prostaglandins which originate from the contact between the embolus and the pulmonary artery endothelium are also possibly involved in the response to PE.

PE increases pulmonary arterial resistance and pulmonary arterial pressure and therefore the work of the right ventricle. Symptoms and signs are related both to the extent of arterial obstruction and to the pre-embolic state of the cardiovascular system. When there are no pre-existing cardiopulmonary problems, the degree of cardiovascular impairment is proportional to the magnitude of the arterial obstruction. However, if there is chronic cardiorespiratory impairment, even a limited PE may be fatal or cause severe disturbance with major symptoms and signs.

DIAGNOSIS The symptoms and signs of PE may be similar to those of other cardiorespiratory diseases. Dyspnoea (75% of patients) and tachypnoea are frequent clinical observations and the former is often associated with chest pain (75%). Haemoptysis (25%) in association with pleural friction rub (8–10%), gallop rhythm, cyanosis (10%) and chest splinting are present together in only a fifth and the triad dyspnoea–chest pain–haemoptysis in 15%. Chest pain (frequent with massive emboli but rarely described with small emboli) is often described as a dull, substernal tightness. Clinical features of deep venous thrombosis are found in 33% of patients but, when non-invasive investigations (duplex or colour-duplex scanning) are used, this figure rises to 45%. Tachypnoea and tachycardia, often not persistent, are the most common findings. Tachycardia is present in 60% and 10% have an accentuated P_2 on the electrocardiogram. Marked tachycardia and tachypnoea indicate massive embolism. In severe right ventricular dysfunction, wide, almost fixed splitting of the second heart sound is a bad prognostic sign. An altered mental state is observed in 20–30% of patients. Because the lower lobes are the most frequent location, a friction rub is most likely to be heard there. Clinical evidence of bronchoconstriction is often present. An increase in temperature (37.5–38.5°C (100–101°F)) is a common finding.

LABORATORY AND INVESTIGATIVE FINDINGS

Blood tests

Variations in serum enzyme concentrations may be indicative of PE but are not diagnostic. Elevation of lactic dehydrogenase (LDH) and bilirubin concentrations with a normal serum glutamate-oxaloacetate transaminase (SGOT) may be present but in massive PE with acute cardiovascular changes this triad is not diagnostic. Changes in the blood require some time to develop and therefore diagnostic methods which detect PE at an earlier stage are desirable.

Arterial blood gas analysis can be useful but hypoxaemia is often variable in patients with a PE. An underperfused segment of lung may marginally increase delivery of un-oxygenated blood to the left side of the heart but a low arterial PO_2 may indicate only massive embolism which is threatening life.

Electrocardiography

About 10–15% of patients with PE have acute electrocardiographic changes. Common abnormalities are T-wave inversion and ST-segment depression, the result of myocardial ischaemia from decreased cardiac output and coronary arterial pressure, and increased right ventricular pressure. Usually the electrocardiographic changes have to be regarded as non-specific.

Imaging

An initial chest x-ray is usually normal in that the pathophysiological changes should not be expected to produce alterations in radiodensity. There is usually no evidence of congestion. The peripheral lung fields are if anything more radiolucent but it is difficult to pick up such evidence of underperfusion without considerable experience (**Figure 7.1**). Later, typical wedge-shaped peripheral infiltrates may appear. An effusion may also develop if the lung is infarcted and the pleura consequently inflamed.

A definitive diagnosis from imaging can only be made by pulmonary angiography though a preliminary radioisotope perfusion scan that shows the distribution of pulmonary artery blood flow and underperfused areas in the lung fields is helpful in deciding which patients should be subject to angiography. A perfusion scan

a

b

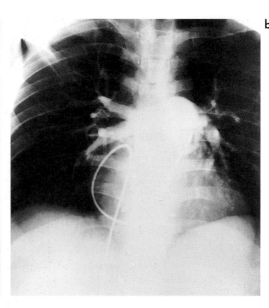

Figure 7.1
(a) Chest x-ray and
(b) pulmonary
angiogram of a
patient with extensive
pulmonary emboli
involving both lungs.
Note that (a) shows
only some atelectatic
changes in the right
lower lobe.

is done by the intravenous injection of albumin-labelled with technetium (^{99m}Tc) or iodine (^{131}I) and should show a radiolucent area of underperfusion (**Figure 7.2**). However, lesions present before a possible embolic event, such as pneumonitis, atelectasis, emphysematous bullae or neoplasm, regularly demonstrate a defect on scan and so produce a false-positive image. Therefore, such abnormal areas must if possible be excluded by a simultaneous plain chest x-ray or a ventilation scan (see below) or both. The pulmonary perfusion scan is considered useful in substantiating the clinical impression of pulmonary embolism before treatment is begun.

Scanning can also be repeated with minimal discomfort to the patient and is the best means of following the evolution of PE. A perfusion scan with multiple segmental or lobar defects is interpreted as *high probability*, whereas subsegmental or non-segmental perfusion defects are considered *low probability* for PE (**Figure 7.3**).

Figure 7.2 Pulmonary
perfusion/ventilation
scans indicative of
pulmonary embolism.

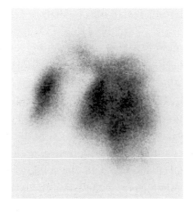

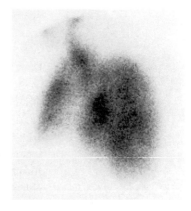

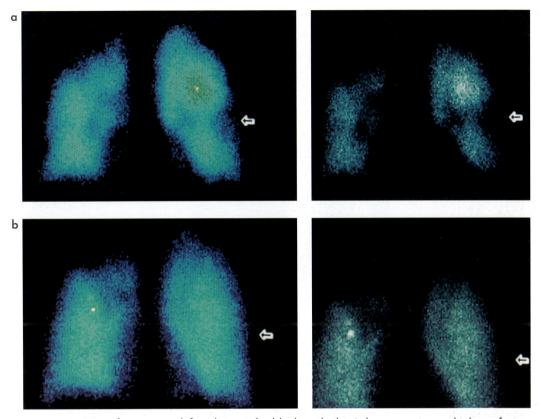

Figure 7.3 (a) Perfusion scan (left: colour; right: black and white) demonstrating multiple perfusion defect in both lungs. Arrow points to peripheral segmental defect indicative of a high probability of previous pulmonary embolism. No defect is shown on ventilation scan in this region.
(b) Ventilation scan (left: colour; right: black and white). Perfusion and ventilation defect shown in left apex indicate that this segment is consolidated (cause unknown).

[133]Xenon ventilation scanning increases the sensitivity of perfusion scans because it differentiates underperfused and underventilated areas by providing information about the distribution of the inhaled gas. Typically PE causes perfusion defects in an area of normal ventilation. However, perfusion defects are often associated with ventilation defects. PE is present in about 90% of patients with a high probability perfusion scan and a mismatch on combined scanning between ventilation and perfusion.

Angiography   Selective pulmonary arteriography is the only definitive method to establish the diagnosis. The potential serious nature of the disease and the significant risks of treatment justify the use of angiography whenever the diagnosis is in reasonable doubt. Arteriography performed within 48 hours of the clinical episode is extremely reliable. The diagnosis is established by the demonstration of unequiv-

Figure 7.4 Right lower pulmonary artery angiogram with a filling defect clearly seen and an associated hypoperfusion of the lower lobe of the lung. These are classical signs of pulmonary embolism.

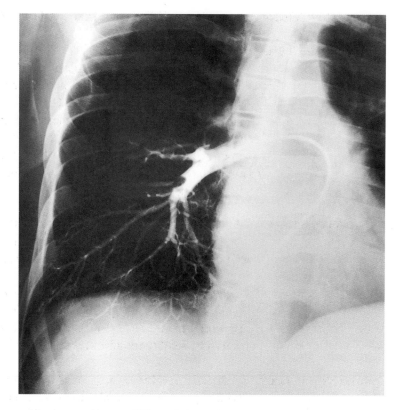

ocal obstruction or filling defects in the pulmonary arterial tree (**Figure 7.4**). Lobar segmental branches are occluded most often but occasionally total obstruction of a main pulmonary artery is found and is usually associated with the most severe symptoms.

DIFFERENTIAL DIAGNOSIS

All forms of embarrassment to cardiac function such as myocardial infarction, congestive heart failure, angina pectoris and aortic dissection may produce clinical features and electrocardiographic changes that can be confused with PE. Respiratory conditions which cause acute respiratory distress—acute pneumonia, lung collapse and pneumothorax—may also cause confusion. Pain which can resemble that encountered in PE may be caused by viral pleuritis or pericarditis. Pulmonary lesions which can mimic the imaging appearances of PE, if a chest x-ray has not been taken before the incident, include lung abscess, tuberculosis and pulmonary neoplasm.

Both the acute onset of atrial fibrillation in a patient without pre-existing cardiac disease, and a sudden deterioration in cardiac function in a patient known to have cardiac disease likely to produce congestive heart failure, suggest the possibility of PE.

PREVENTION Prophylaxis of PE is considered in Chapter 8.

MANAGEMENT *Medical treatment*
The patient's limbs should be elevated to increase the rate of venous blood flow and kept in this position provided this does not cause cardiorespiratory distress. Graduated compression stockings have the same effect and both measures may decrease the rate of growth of the thrombus and limit the size of a potential embolus. In massive pulmonary embolism with hypotension, the usual medical measures directed towards restoring perfusion are used—vasopressors and inotropic agents.

Anticoagulation After an intravenous bolus of heparin (10 000 units in an adult), heparin is administered by continuous intravenous infusion (1000–2000 units/hour) for 7–10 days (see pp. 172–173 for details). Oral anticoagulants are started as soon as the general condition of the patient and the particular circumstances permit. Heparin is discontinued 4 5 days after a one-stage prothrombin time of 1.3 – 1.5 times the control (INR 2 to 3) has been obtained. Oral anticoagulants are usually continued for a period of 3 – 6 months.

Thrombolytic therapy Urokinase combined with heparin significantly accelerates the lysis of pulmonary thromboemboli at 24 hours by comparison with heparin alone. However, significant differences in clinical outcome have not been observed. Nevertheless thrombolysis is indicated in severely ill patients in shock or with right heart failure as well as for those with severe pulmonary hypertension who may die if a further PE occurs.

  The following regimens are used and are equally effective:

♦ *urokinase:* an initial dose of 4400 IU/kg intravenously followed by 4400 IU/kg per hour for 12 hours;
♦ *streptokinase:* 250 000 IU intravenously in 30 minutes, followed by 100 000 IU/h for 24 hours;
♦ *alteplase:* (recombinant tissue plasminogen activator) 90 – 100 mg intravenously over 7 hours.

Heparin is always administered after the thrombolytic infusion.

Complications Bleeding is the most common complication of thrombolytic treatment and can occur into accidental or surgical wounds, at sites of catheterization and into areas that have been involved in a recent stroke. Therefore lytic treatment should not be used within 3 weeks of such events. Streptokinase is also pyrogenic and may cause allergic reactions.

Surgery Operation to remove emboli from the pulmonary artery directly can be life-saving in selected patients with massive embolism. The principal indication for pulmonary embolectomy is severe, refractory hypotension after resuscitation in subjects with massive embolism proved by lung scan or pulmonary arteriogram and who have not made a response to or have contraindications to the use of thrombolytic therapy. Such circumstances are rare: most patients previously thought to require embolectomy now respond favourably to heparinization, vasopressors and inotropic agents.

Open surgery is now performed using cardiopulmonary bypass. In many patients more than half of the pulmonary arterial system is occluded but exceptions are those with pre-existing cardiac or respiratory insufficiency. A survival rate of 75–80% may be obtained.

Transvenous embolectomy Large suction catheters are inserted through the femoral vein and directed to the embolus under angiographic control. The technique is now used more frequently than open surgery to remove life-

Figure 7.5
A Greenfield filter placed in the infrarenal vena cava in an elderly lady with recurrent pulmonary embolization from an extensive iliofemoral vein thrombosis.

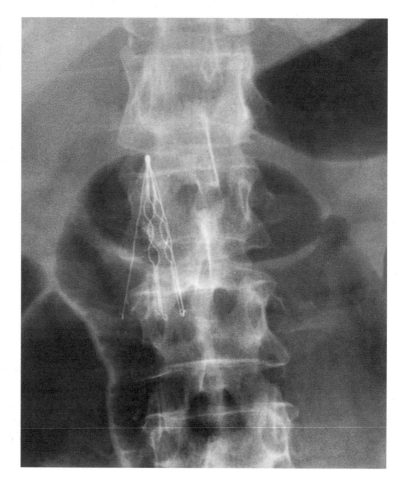

threatening pulmonary emboli. Catheter-based methods are much simpler, more cost-effective, less stressful and dangerous and can directly follow an angiographic diagnosis. A catheter in the pulmonary artery also allows the direction of thrombolysis at residual clot and a caval filter (**Figure 7.5**) can be inserted. All these advantages over open operation make the use of transvenous embolectomy the now preferred technique.

Treatment at the site of origin   Either surgical treatment or local thrombolysis are occasionally used to prevent the genesis of further emboli from a known site.

PROGNOSIS   Only 10–12% of those who sustain a symptomatic episode die within an hour. About 30% of undiagnosed or untreated patients die, the majority as a result of recurrent embolism. That most patients survive an initial PE is because, as the embolus is small, the initial pulmonary arterial obstruction is limited and *in situ* lysis is rapid. In patients who survive long enough for the diagnosis to be established and who then receive adequate therapy, death is relatively uncommon. Age affects the outlook: in the young, appropriately diagnosed and managed, the prognosis of PE is good; in the elderly and sick the prognosis is less satisfactory and mainly determined by concomitant disorders.

After a PE, progressive resolution of obstruction by lysis and macrophage removal of clot is usually apparent within a few weeks but can be detected in most patients by lung scanning or arteriography within a few days of the initial episode. Complete resolution of the obstruction is usual and the only final evidence of a previous lesion may be moderate thickening of the endothelium at the embolic site. The haemodynamic improvement depends on the quality of reperfusion of the pulmonary vascular segment.

The prognosis in the immediate aftermath of an embolus is generally determined by the presence of associated clinical conditions (mainly cardiac and respiratory insufficiency). Extensive and repeated pulmonary emboli produce pulmonary hypertension with right heart failure (cor pulmonale) which is refractory to treatment.

BIBLIOGRAPHY

Anderson DR, Levine MN. Thrombolytic therapy for the treatment of acute pulmonary embolism. *Can Med Assoc J* 1992; **146:** 1317.

Benotti JR, Dalen JE. The natural history of pulmonary embolism. *Clin Chest Med* 1984; **5:** 403.

Biello DR. Radiological (scintigraphic) evaluation of patients with suspected pulmonary thromboembolism. *JAMA* 1987; **257**: 3257.

Goldhaber SZ *et al.* Randomised controlled trial of recombinant tissue plasminogen activator versus urokinase in the treatment of acute pulmonary embolism. *Lancet* 1988; **2**: 203.

Goldstone J. Veins and lymphatics. In: Way LW, ed. *Current Surgical Diagnosis and Treatment.* 10th ed. East Norwalk, USA: Appleton and Lange, 1994;783.

Harley DP *et al.* Pulmonary embolism secondary to venous thrombosis of the arm. *Am J Surg* 1984; **147**: 221.

Hull RD *et al.* Pulmonary embolism in outpatients with pleuritic chest pain. *Arch Intern Med* 1988; **148**: 838.

Marder VJ, Sherry S. Thrombolytic therapy: current status (2 parts). *N Engl J Med* 1988; **318**: 1512 & 1585.

Mattox KL *et al.* Pulmonary embolectomy for acute massive pulmonary embolism. *Ann Surg* 1982; **195**: 726.

Moran KT, Jewell ER, Persson AV. The role of thrombolytic therapy in surgical practice. *Br J Surg* 1989; **76**: 298.

PIOPED Investigators. Value of ventilation/perfusion scan in acute pulmonary embolism: the prospective investigation of pulmonary embolism diagnosis. *JAMA* 1990; **263**: 2753.

Rosenthal D *et al.* Massive pulmonary embolism: triple-armed therapy. *J Vasc Surg* 1989; **9**: 261.

Schwarz F *et al.* Sustained improvement of pulmonary hemodynamics in patients at rest and during exercise after thrombolytic treatment of massive pulmonary embolism. *Circulation* 1985; **71**: 117.

West JW. Pulmonary embolism. *Med Clin North Am* 1986; **70**: 877.

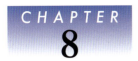

Prevention of venous thromboembolism

THE PROBLEM AND NEED FOR PREVENTION

Deep venous thrombosis (DVT) and pulmonary embolism (PE) are major health problems with two serious outcomes. The first, as described in Chapters 6 and 11, is the precursor of chronic venous insufficiency. The second may be immediately fatal and, in the long term, carries the risk of development of pulmonary hypertension from recurrent embolism. Both have a great impact on health care costs. The yearly rate of DVT is around 160 per 100 000 in the general population, the rate of fatal PE is 60 and the number of venous ulcers 200. However, the proportion of ulceration stemming from a previous DVT is still unknown.

The attitudes and beliefs about prophylaxis show great regional and specialist variations. This is true for the definition of risk groups, the proportion of patients who receive prophylaxis and the prophylactic method that is chosen.

ASSESSMENT OF RISK OF THROMBOEMBOLISM

It is possible, using clinical criteria based on extensive studies of asymptomatic and symptomatic DVT and PE, to categorize patients into risk groups. The useful procedure for determining whether or not to use prophylaxis and the form it should take, is to assign patients, using clinical criteria, to one of three classes: *high, medium* or *low* risk. Categorization in this manner for surgical, obstetric and gynaecological, and medical patients is given in **Tables 8.1, 8.2** and **8.3**.

Table 8.1 Risk categories in surgical patients (risk assessed by objective tests)

Risk category	Calf-vein thrombosis (%)	Proximal-vein thrombosis (%)	Fatal PE (%)
High General and urological surgery in patients >40 years with recent history of DVT or PE Extensive pelvic or abdominal surgery for malignant disease Major orthopaedic surgery of lower limbs	40–80	10–30	1–5
Moderate General surgery in patients >40 years and lasting 30 min or more in patients <40 years on oral contraceptives	10–40	2–10	0.1–0.7
Low Uncomplicated surgery in patients <40 years without additional risk factors Minor surgery (<30 min) in patients >40years without additional risk factors	<10	<1	<0.01

Table 8.2 Risk categories in gynaecology and obstetrics

	Gynaecology	Obstetrics*
High risk	History of previous DVT/PE Age >60 Cancer Thrombophilic condition	History of previous DVT/PE
Moderate risk	Patients >40 years undergoing major surgery Patients <40 years on oral contraceptives undergoing major surgery	Thrombophilic condition Patients >40 years
Low risk	Uncomplicated surgery in patients <40 years without additional risk factors Minor surgery (<30 min) Patients >40 years without additional risk factors	

* The risk of DVT in obstetric patients with pre-eclampsia and other risk factors is unknown but prophylaxis should be considered.

Table 8.3 Risk categories in medical patients

High risk
  Stroke
  Congestive heart failure
  Thrombophilia with additional disease
Moderate/low risk
  All immobilized patients with active disease (the risk is increased by infectious diseases, malignancy, and other risk factors)

THE PATIENTS

Surgical patients

Those who sustain major trauma or undergo operative procedures without anticoagulation are at risk of developing venous thrombo-embolism. The degree of risk is increased by the different factors indicated in **Table 8.4**. These factors are further modified by the individual procedure (**Table 8.5**) and the management associated with it, including operative duration, type of anaesthesia, pre- and postoperative immobility, level of hydration and the presence of sepsis.

Table 8.4 Factors increasing the risk of venous thrombosis

Abnormal vein wall
  Varicose veins
  Previous DVT
  Trauma to vein walls (cannulation)
  Inflammatory process around the veins
  (especially pelvic)
Reduced venous flow
  Bed rest
  Prolonged incorrect position (leg dependency)
  Restriction of leg motion (cast, paralysis, postoperative pain)
  Congestive heart failure
  Extrinsic compression of veins (tumours)
  External compression (pillow, bandages)
  Decreased arterial flow (shock)
Hypercoagulability
  Trauma (surgery, childbirth, injury)
  Hyperviscosity
  Tumours
  Hormones, contraceptives
  Deficiency of protein C, protein S and antithrombin III

Table 8.5 Risk groups in trauma and surgery in order of decreasing frequency of DVT

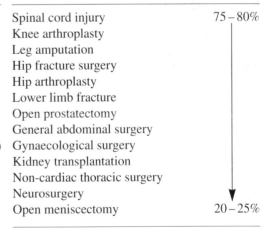

Spinal cord injury	75–80%
Knee arthroplasty	
Leg amputation	
Hip fracture surgery	
Hip arthroplasty	
Lower limb fracture	
Open prostatectomy	
General abdominal surgery	
Gynaecological surgery	
Kidney transplantation	
Non-cardiac thoracic surgery	
Neurosurgery	
Open meniscectomy	20–25%

Gynaecological and obstetric patients

The reported overall incidence of thromboembolic complications in gynaecological patients undergoing surgery is similar to that observed in general surgery. Pulmonary embolism is a leading cause of death following operation for gynaecological cancer. In pregnancy, DVT occurs in 0.13–0.5/1000 in the antepartum period and 0.61–1.5/1000 in postpartum patients. PE is an important cause of maternal mortality.

Risk factors associated with DVT include those already mentioned. In addition, others associated with DVT/PE in pregnancy are caesarean section, advanced maternal age and thrombophilic states. There is an increased risk of venous thrombosis in women taking oral contraceptives which contain greater than 50 μg of oestrogen. However, there are no data on the low dose oral contraceptives currently in use.

Medical patients

There is less information available on medical as distinct from surgical patients. However, an increased risk of venous thromboembolism has been shown in patients with acute myocardial infarction, cerebrovascular accidents and in those who are immobilized for medical reasons.

PREDISPOSING HAEMATOLOGICAL CAUSES

Thrombophilia

Thrombophilia (congenital or acquired predisposition to thrombosis) is rare but should be seriously considered in patients defined as having had a documented but unexplained thrombotic episode below the age of 40, recurrent DVTs or a positive family history. The frequency of congenital thrombophilia in consecutive patients with confirmed thrombosis is approximately 8%. In addition, a number of acquired haematological abnormalities are associated with a predisposition to venous thromboembolism (e.g. lupus anticoagulant, anticardiolipin, myeloproliferative disease).

The recommended screening sequences are:

♦ *General:* complete blood count including platelets.
♦ *Suspected congenital thrombophilia:* antithrombin III, protein C, protein S, fibrinogen/thrombin clotting time.
♦ *Suspected acquired thrombophilia:* activated partial thromboplastin time (APTT) and anticardiolipin antibody.

Fibrinolysis

Normal levels of plasminogen, plasminogen and prourokinase activator inhibitor activity, tissue plasminogen activator activity, pre- and post-stress lysis may be considered to rule out an abnormality in the fibrinolytic system if the above tests are normal. However, the clinical relevance of abnormalities in the fibrinolytic system is uncertain.

Management

Patients with confirmed congenital thrombophilia should be considered at high risk for thromboembolism. In those who have symptoms, the duration of treatment is uncertain and should be considered case by case, taking into account the benefit–risk ratio for the individual. In asymptomatic patients the value of primary prophylaxis is not yet known but protection is needed during surgery or the course of any medical condition associated with an increased risk of thrombosis.

Pregnant women with thrombophilia are a special subgroup at risk throughout pregnancy and should be considered for prophylaxis. The period of risk begins early in the first trimester, particularly in those with antithrombin III deficiency.

Acquired haematological abnormalities

The decision about primary prophylaxis should be made on an individual basis.

ORAL OESTROGEN CONTRACEPTION AND PREDISPOSITION TO VENOUS THROMBOSIS

There is epidemiological evidence to suggest a relationship between oestrogen-containing oral contraceptives and venous thromboembolism. Therefore, the oral contraceptive pill is contraindicated in patients with other predisposing causes of thromboembolism.

The use of combination oral contraceptives may also be associated with increased risk of DVT in patients undergoing gynaecological surgery.

SCREENING FOR THROMBOEMBOLISM

Routine screening for asymptomatic pulmonary emboli is neither necessary nor cost-effective. It is well documented that the majority of pulmonary emboli and the majority of fatal pulmonary emboli take place after an asymptomatic DVT. The implication of this finding is that, in epidemiological work on incidence, it is important to use an investigation which will detect all peripheral thrombi. In *low- and medium-risk patients* who are protected by a proven prophylactic method, routine screening for DVT is not needed. In *high-risk patients,* even with established methods of prophylaxis, the incidence of asymptomatic DVT is considerable and screening may be beneficial.

Practical methods for screening high-risk patients are B-mode ultrasound and duplex and colour-duplex scanning. However, the simple continuous-wave Doppler is not very reliable, particularly if the thrombosis has not produced complete obstruction in an axial vein. B-mode ultrasound and, better, colour-duplex scanning (which is faster and more precise) are good alternatives to venography which is more expensive and is associated with more complications.

PROPHYLAXIS   *General surgery and urology*

Graduated compression stockings have been shown to be effective in reducing the incidence of DVT in patients younger than 45 years old and at mild to moderate risk. Intermittent pneumatic compression (IPC) is also effective. There is not enough information to evaluate other methods of mechanical prophylaxis. Further, there is little evidence that antiplatelet agents are effective in reducing the incidence of thromboembolism and also there are insufficient data to support the use of oral anticoagulants for primary prophylaxis. Dextran has been shown to be effective in reducing fatal pulmonary embolism—though the evidence that it also reduces the incidence of DVT is weak—but has risks of fluid overload and can produce anaphylactic reactions.

By interfering with the immune complex formation (hapten inhibition) it is possible to counteract dextran reactions.

Low-dose conventional heparin and low-molecular-weight heparins (LMWH) are effective in reducing both DVT and PE in general surgical patients but heparinoids have been insufficiently studied.

Combinations of mechanical and pharmacological methods may be more effective than either used alone.

As already described, patients can be classified into *low, medium* and *high risk* of developing thromboembolism. *Low-risk patients* may receive prophylaxis but the data objectively to support this approach as mandatory are not available. However, graduated compression stockings, which are simple to use and inexpensive, should be considered. For *medium-risk patients,* low-dose heparin or LMWH are effective and should be used, preferably in combination with graduated stockings. An alternative recommendation may be IPC used continuously and also combined with stockings until the patient is ambulant. *High-risk patients* must receive aggressive prophylaxis on the same lines as those at medium risk.

Whenever it is used, prophylaxis should be initiated preoperatively and continued for 7–10 days. This period should be extended if hospital stay is prolonged or the risk continues. For women taking oral contraceptive agents, if these cannot be stopped 4–6 weeks before surgery, consideration should be given to increasing the intensity of prophylaxis. Patients with a high risk of bleeding, either from a known coagulation disorder or because of a specific surgical procedures, are better treated with mechanical methods.

Neurosurgery Mechanical methods are the only ones appropriate: graduated stockings and IPC.

Orthopaedic surgery and trauma Patients undergoing both elective and emergency operations are at a high risk of developing postoperative DVT/PE. Total hip replacement without prophylaxis is associated with a high incidence of DVT (about 50%) and of PE of which 1–3% are fatal. The high incidence of DVT carries the additional problem of later development of chronic venous insufficiency, the incidence of which has been estimated to be approximately 50% at 5 years after an episode of DVT. These observations emphasize the need to protect such high risk patients by routine prophylaxis.

Methods of prophylaxis which have been used in this group include aspirin, dextran, fixed low-dose unfractionated heparin (FLDUH), adjusted dose heparin, addition of dihydroergotamine to FLDUH, fixed mini-dose or full dose of oral anticoagulant therapy, external pneumatic compression, LMWH and some heparinoids. The following recommendations are made.

Elective surgery There is insufficient evidence to recommend antiplatelet drugs for prophylaxis. Dextran is only moderately effective and has inherent risks (see above). Fixed low-dose unfractionated heparin prophylaxis (5000 units twice or three times a day) is moderately effective but increasing the dosage enhances the bleeding risk. Adjusting the heparin dosage to the results of a coagulation assay is more effective but difficult to manage. The addition of dihydroergotamine (DHE) to FLDUH enhances effectiveness but has the inherent risk of vasospasm. Adjusting the dose of oral anticoagulants to a desired international normalized ratio (INR, see p. 82) improves efficacy but is more complex to manage. IPC with and without graduated stockings works but has some practical limitations. Fixed dose LMWH is very effective. The information on heparinoids is limited but encouraging and the dose, efficacy and safety of each product need to be assessed separately.

Prophylaxis should be started preoperatively and continued for 7–10 days or until the patient is fully ambulant. Experience with fixed low-dose heparin indicates that there is no evidence that preoperative prophylaxis increases the risk of haemorrhage associated with spinal or epidural anaesthesia.

A limited number of studies are available for patients undergoing knee replacement. Results do not permit a firm recommendation but the modalities effective in patients undergoing hip replacement can also be applied to the knee.

Emergency surgery   The methods to be used for hip and other major fractures are comparable to those for elective hip surgery and should be started as soon as possible. DHE/heparin is contraindicated.

Obstetrics and gynaecology   *Gynaecological surgery*
Low-risk patients may receive prophylaxis on an individual basis. Graduated stockings should be considered. Moderate-risk patients are treated with low-dose heparin (5000 units twice daily). IPC should also be considered in that it has been shown to be valuable in higher-risk patients. Dextran and warfarin are not recommended for routine prophylaxis but may have a role when LDH is contraindicated. LMWH is also effective but data on the use of graduated stockings in moderate-risk gynaecological surgery are insufficient. Discontinuation of oral contraceptives 4–6 weeks before surgery should be considered. If oral contraceptives have not been discontinued, prophylaxis should be provided.

In high-risk patients, low-dose heparin (5000 units every 8 hours), LMWH or IPC used continuously for at least 5 days, provides effective prophylaxis. Combined methods and extension of the period of prophylaxis for extended periods require better definition. Data evaluating graduated stockings for high-risk gynaecological patients do not permit precise evaluation.

Pregnancy   Low-dose heparin prophylaxis is commonly used in pregnant patients at high risk of DVT and pulmonary embolism though data from controlled trials are lacking. There is also insufficient information on either the optimum timing or dose schedule of low-dose heparin. Oral anticoagulants are contraindicated in the first trimester because of the risk of damage to the fetus; the available data indicate that they are also associated with fetal abnormalities in the second trimester and increased maternal–fetal bleeding in both the second and third trimesters. The benefits of prophylaxis have not been clearly demonstrated in patients undergoing caesarean section who have no additional risk factors. Perioperative and postpartum prophylaxis should be seriously considered in the presence of additional risk factors.

There are still only limited data on the use of LMWH or mechanical methods in pregnancy. Women who develop DVT with or without a PE during pregnancy should be treated with therapeutic levels of heparin continued throughout the duration of pregnancy, labour and delivery. Anticoagulation is usually continued for at least 4–6 weeks postpartum though the optimal duration of therapy has yet to be established.

The development of deep vein thrombosis or pulmonary embolus during pregnancy is an indication for haematological screening to detect thrombophilia.

Medical patients   *Acute myocardial infarction*
Patients who do not receive anticoagulant therapy as part of their primary treatment are at risk of venous thromboembolism. The recommended prophylaxis is low-dose heparin or LMWH.

Stroke   Patients with ischaemic stroke are at high risk. The recommended prophylaxis is either low-dose heparin, LMWH or low-molecular-weight heparinoid.

Immobilized general medical patients   Those considered at risk should receive prophylaxis. The following can be considered: graduated compression stockings; intermittent pneumatic compression; low-dose heparin; LMWH; low-molecular-weight heparinoid; oral anticoagulants.

COMBINED FORMS OF PROPHYLAXIS   *Surgery*
High-risk patients
Apart from single regimens that have been demonstrated to be effective and safe, such as low-dose heparin and LMWH, combinations may be considered for use by individual surgical teams depending on their case mix and resources. Options are low-dose heparin or LMWH combined with mechanical methods.

Moderate-risk patients   Combined mechanical methods may be applied as an alternative to low-dose heparin or LMWH.

Gynaecology and obstetrics   Combinations of prophylaxis have not been adequately evaluated but on the basis of results of surgical trials, combined prophylaxis should be considered.

General medicine   In high-risk patients there is a lack of studies that have used combined methods. Hence, specific recommendations cannot be made.

COST-EFFECTIVENESS OF PREVENTION IN ALL GROUPS

In discussing prophylactic methods used in the prevention of thromboembolism, it is important to consider health economics. Primary prevention is more cost-effective than secondary prevention undertaken by routine screening of postoperative patients. In *medium- and high-risk patients*, the costs following thromboembolism are so high that the currently recommended methods of primary prophylaxis are very cost-effective. In *low-risk patients* no data are available at present concerning the cost-effectiveness of the current recommended prophylactic methods.

SECONDARY PREVENTION

The objectives of treatment of thromboembolism are to prevent extension of thrombus which may lead both to local effects and to pulmonary embolus. The first are commonly destruction of the valves in the deep veins with the long-term development of chronic venous insufficiency and, rarely, progression, because of raised intracompartment pressure, to phlegmasia cerulea dolens, venous gangrene and limb loss. The second may be a single fatal or non-fatal event or repeated with the ultimate development of chronic pulmonary hypertension.

Anticoagulants are discussed in Chapter 6. In summary, initial treatment is with heparin, preferably by continuous intravenous administration and followed immediately or after the lapse of a few days by conversion to oral anticoagulation. The latter should be continued for a period of at least 3 months in patients with a first episode of venous thrombosis and no persistent risk factors. However, the optimal duration of therapy is not known. Patients with a recurrent episode of venous thrombosis should be treated with heparin with a similar therapeutic regimen as for patients with a first episode of DVT but it is not clear for how long treatment should continue. Adjusted doses of subcutaneous heparin may be used as secondary prophylaxis in special clinical conditions such as pregnancy and other contraindications to oral anticoagulant therapy.

LMWHs given subcutaneously have been shown to be as effective as standard heparin for the initial treatment of DVTs judged by the reduction of the thrombus size measured by repeated venography. Preliminary results demonstrate that LMWHs are as effective as adjusted dose intravenous standard heparin in the prevention of symptomatic recurrent venous thromboembolism during long-term follow-up. There is good evidence that *thrombolytic therapy* produces a more effective lysis in proximal DVT than does unfractionated heparin but its use is limited because the benefit–risk ratio of this treatment as compared with unfractionated heparin has not yet been established. Therefore, there is at present insufficient evidence that all patients with DVT should receive thrombolytic therapy; it may be considered, in the absence of contraindications, for selected patients who suffer from recent massive vein thrombosis.

Thrombectomy (Chapter 6) is indicated to save a limb threatened by venous gangrene but its use in other circumstances has been limited and exact indications have not been established.

Caval filters (Chapter 7) are indicated when anticoagulation is contraindicated in the management of either pulmonary embolism or venous thrombosis above the knee or when adequate anticoagulation fails to prevent recurrent thromboembolism. For thrombosis extending to or involving the renal veins and in pregnant patients, a device shown by prospective trials to be effective (such as a Greenfield filter) should be placed above the level of the renal veins. Extended indications for filter insertion are under clinical investigation.

PROBLEMS WHICH REMAIN TO BE EVALUATED

◆ The risk of DVT/PE may continue beyond the patient's hospital stay and has not been assessed by a prospective trial.

◆ There is an urgent need for a proper randomized study to compare prophylactic methods started before or after operation.

◆ The comparative efficacy in patients at moderate risk of fixed low-dose heparin and LMWH, as judged by prevention of PE and overall mortality, requires study.

◆ Further studies are required to see whether graduated stockings and/or IPC enhance the efficacy of pharmacological methods.

◆ A prospective analysis, based on the establishment of a register, of the prevalence of haemorrhage in patients who have a spinal or epidural anaesthetic and who have also received prophylaxis with anticoagulants should be undertaken.

◆ There is an urgent need to establish the risk of DVT in large series of the new minimally invasive abdominal surgical procedures.

◆ There is an urgent need for a multicentre trial to compare standard heparin with LMWH in high-risk pregnant patients for their efficacy, safety and side effects such as osteoporosis.

BIBLIOGRAPHY

Bergqvist D, Comerota A, Nicolaides AN, Scurr J, eds. *Prevention of Venous Thromboembolism*. European Workshop and Consensus Statement. London: Med-Orion, 1994.

Superficial thrombophlebitis

GENERAL CONSIDERATIONS

Superficial thrombophlebitis is a poorly studied and often neglected clinical condition commonly seen in older patients. Causes of thrombophlebitis in superficial veins include:

◆ varicose veins;
◆ mechanical or chemical trauma usually from intravenous therapy;
◆ radiation injury;
◆ bacterial or fungal infections;
◆ haematologial disorders;
◆ immune reactions.

In the upper extremities drug misuse and catheters inserted for diagnostic or therapeutic purposes are common causes. The condition is a clinical entity and manifests itself as a painful, tender, swollen vein often with some perivenous signs of inflammation and progressing to a thrombosed channel which can be felt as an initially tender 'cord' in the line of the vein.

PATHOLOGICAL FEATURES

Although the condition appears to be inflammatory in nature, the background is usually not obviously one of infection. Thrombophlebitis often develops after minor trauma to a varicose vein, usually along the course of an incompetent long saphenous vein (**Figure 9.1**). The thrombus adheres to the vein wall and propagates proximally or distally as a clot often without inflammatory features. The leading edge of this extension may occasionally

Figure 9.1 and Figure 9.2 Thrombophlebitis of the long saphenous vein and extension of the proximal thrombus into the femoral vein at the saphenofemoral junction (arrow).

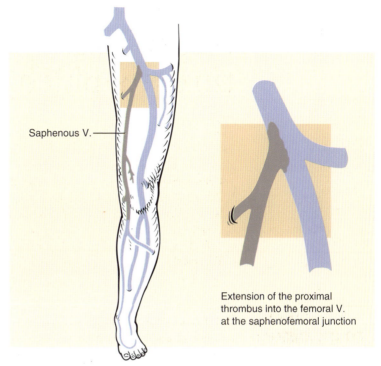

Saphenous V.

Extension of the proximal thrombus into the femoral V. at the saphenofemoral junction

extend into the deep venous system directly, for example at the saphenofemoral junction (**Figure 9.2**) or through an incompetent perforating vein. Detachment can then occur with pulmonary embolus though this event is rare. Furthermore, in that the embolus is usually small, cardiorespiratory symptoms and signs are very rarely observed. However, it must be stressed that a deep venous thrombosis and a pulmonary embolus *can* result from an acute attack of superficial thrombophlebitis and there is the possibility that the embolus may be infected. In some instances the valves in the deep system may be destroyed and chronic venous insufficiency (Chapter 11) results.

NATURAL HISTORY Most attacks resolve spontaneously with elevation of the affected limb supplemented, in circumstances where there is infection, by antibiotic therapy. As noted above, progression to deep venous thrombosis, pulmonary embolization and postphlebitic syndrome may rarely occur. Depending on the extent of the process, the inflammatory reaction usually takes between 2 and 6 weeks to subside but the thrombosed vein may remain tender and palpable for many months. In patients with superficial varicosities, recurrence is frequent either in the same vein or in other segments of the superficial system.

DIAGNOSIS

In varicose veins the process most commonly involves the long saphenous vein and its tributaries and tends to remain localized. Thrombophlebitis is often seen in patients whose varicosities are large and pregnancy is an additional factor. Diagnosis is usually easy because of the superficial site of the thrombosis. The patient may be febrile and have a leucocytosis. There is local pain with induration, heat, tenderness and redness along the course of the vein. Usually there is no oedema or swelling of the extremity. Occasionally pain and the immobilization that follows may cause differences in the size of the two limbs. The thrombosed veins feel like cords or a chain of nodules which are warm and red in comparison with the surrounding areas. In doubtful instances a simple test to diagnose thrombophlebitis is to elevate the limb. When this does not reduce the volume of the veins as is promptly the case with simple varicose veins (**Figure 9.3**) the veins are thrombosed. The extent and spread of thrombophlebitis can easily be ascertained by thermography but the method is not needed to make a diagnosis.

Non-invasive investigations are generally used in most cases of superficial thrombophlebitis to rule out the presence of deep venous thrombosis. Simple B-mode imaging (see Chapter 4) may be employed. It indicates superficial thrombophlebitis when the

Figure 9.3
Incompressible, full veins after leg elevation indicates the presence of superficial thrombophlebitis. The thermographic aspect of this group of superficial thrombosed veins is also shown.

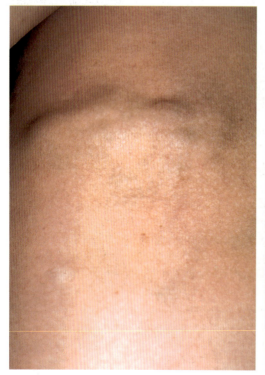
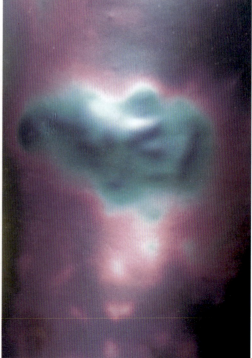

superficial veins (**Figure 9.4**) are not compressible under the ultrasound probe. B-mode scanning is useful to define the level and extent of the superficial thrombus, to confirm that there has not been extension through the deep fascia to the deep system (**Figure 9.4**) and to follow the course of the condition over time.

Invasive investigations such as ascending venography are seldom performed in that ultrasound is efficient.

Figure 9.4
Incompressible veins by B-mode ultrasound.
(a) The presence of a fresh thrombus is indicated by the very low echogenicity of the lumen.
(b) More organized (1–2 weeks old), echogenic thrombus. While the thrombus in (a) can be easily removed by a small incision and squeezing the vein, the echolucent thrombus is more organized and difficult to remove surgically.

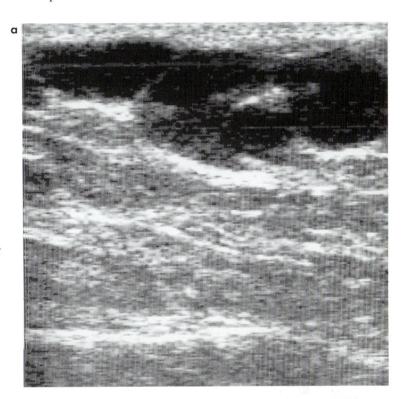

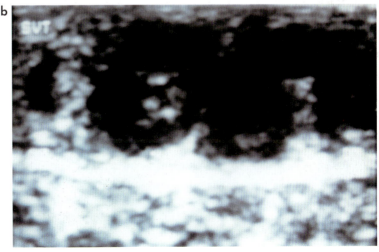

DIFFERENTIAL DIAGNOSIS

In the obese, superficial thrombophlebitis may be confused with cellulitis. A line of redness along the affected vein makes the distinction between the two conditions easier. Other acute inflammatory conditions such as insect bites, erythema nodosum and lymphangitis may be confused with acute superficial thrombophlebitis. Some of the clinical features of superficial thrombophlebitis are, in an extensive case, difficult to distinguish from a deep vein thrombosis especially if there is a difference in the sizes of the two limbs; non-invasive techniques will usually make the distinction clear. In rare instances the two conditions coexist when a superficial phlebitis extends into the deep system via the communicating veins or at the saphenofemoral junction. Chills and high fever suggest infection or suppuration in the involved vein (septic thrombophlebitis). *Staphylococcus aureus* is the microorganism most frequently found but in subjects who abuse drugs almost any pyogenic organism may be present. When the thrombophlebitis is the outcome of intravenous therapy, *Staphylococcus epidermidis* is most usual.

TREATMENT

Non-operative treatment as an outpatient may be used in most minor cases. Treatment is with limb elevation, local heat, analgesics and non-steroidal anti-inflammatory drugs. Patients should be seen every few days to ensure that there is no proximal extension up the thigh or into the deep venous system. Any evidence of this on non-invasive assessment requires inpatient care with initial intravenous heparin followed by oral anticoagulant treatment.

Surgical treatment may be used in patients with recent thrombosis and fresh clots in the veins. Under local anaesthesia, the area containing the superficial clots are incised with a small (No. 11) blade and the clot removed by compressing the vein and squeezing out the thrombus. A compression bandage is applied and elevation used on an outpatient basis. The removal of the thrombus speeds healing and reduces inflammation and pain.

In more severe instances associated with lower limb varicosities and extending above mid-thigh, it is better (in order to avoid the admittedly uncommon event of extension into the deep system and possible pulmonary embolus) to admit the patient at once and operate on the veins on a semi-emergency basis. Ligation and division of the saphenous vein at the saphenofemoral junction and removal of the phlebitic veins and associated tributaries are indicated. Any extension of the thrombus into the common femoral vein should be removed via the opening of the long saphenous vein at the saphenofemoral junction. Thrombophlebitis of the short saphenous vein should likewise be managed in an aggressive fashion by ligating the short saphenous vein at its entry into the popliteal vein and also removing the affected vein segment.

When the thrombus is infected, the appropriate antibiotic treatment should be given, and the phlebitic segment removed to avoid spread into the bloodstream with an ensuing high risk of septic complications.

SUPERFICIAL THROMBOPHLEBITIS WITHOUT VARICOSE VEINS

Thrombophlebitis migrans, intermittent episodes of thrombosis of short segments of superficial veins in the arm or leg, is a consequence of the hypercoagulable state which sometimes accompanies cancers, usually of the mucin-secreting type. Examples are the body and tail of pancreas, stomach, lung, breast and colon and the phlebitic episodes may long antedate any other clinical manifestations of malignancy. Collagen and myeloproliferative diseases are also sometimes associated with thrombophlebitis. There is also a higher incidence of deep venous thrombosis.

Behçet's syndrome was first described in 1887. It is a multisystem disease of uncertain cause with diverse clinical features which include orogenital ulcerations, scronegative arthritis, manifestations of avascular necrosis, superficial thrombophlebitis, and recurrent iriditis. The Budd–Chiari syndrome (sudden occlusion of the main hepatic veins) may be associated with it.

Buerger's disease (thromboangiitis obliterans) is a segmental obliterative condition of small and medium-size arteries of the extremities in young adults and is strongly associated with cigarette smoking. Up to a third of patients present with recurrent, migratory, superficial thrombophlebitis. However, the threat to life and limb comes from the arterial component of the disease.

Mondor's disease is superficial thrombophlebitis in the upper extremities and especially over the chest wall. As with Buerger's disease, young adults with a history of heavy consumption of tobacco are the usual sufferers. A palpable cord is found in the vicinity of the inflamed vein. There may be an underlying chronic pulmonary infection. The disease runs a self-limiting course and the treatment is symptomatic.

CONCLUSIONS

Most cases of superficial thrombophlebitis resolve spontaneously within a few weeks and with simple symptomatic treatment. Pulmonary embolism is uncommon because inflammation of the vein wall produces adherence of the thrombus to it. In the more severe cases, non-invasive investigations are important to exclude extension of the phlebitis into the deep venous system. Recurrent thrombophlebitis and/or the presence of large varices which may cause new episodes of thrombophlebitis are indications for operation.

BIBLIOGRAPHY

Edwards EA. Migrating thrombophlebitis associated with carcinoma. *N Engl J Med* 1949; **240:** 1031.

Hammond JS, Varas R, Ward CG. Suppurative thrombophlebitis: a new look at a continuing problem. *South Med J* 1988; **81:** 969.

Husni EA, Williams WA. Superficial thrombophlebitis of lower limbs. *Surgery* 1982; **91:** 70.

Sarin S et al. Assessment of stripping the long saphenous vein in the treatment of primary varicose veins. *Br J Surg* 1992; **79:** 889.

Venniker R. Venous insufficiency. *Clinic* 1983;1,7:24.

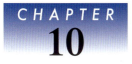

CHAPTER 10

Subclavian and axillary venous thrombosis (SAVT)

GENERAL CONSIDERATIONS

Subclavian and axillary vein thrombosis (SAVT) account for only 1–2% of cases of deep venous thrombosis. This relatively low incidence is thought to be the consequence of the short length of these veins and the relative absence of impediment to blood flow compared with the lower limbs. SAVTs may be classified by cause into three groups (**Table 10.1**).

Table 10.1
Aetiological factors in the pathogenesis of SAVT (C. Fisher)

Iatrogenic
  in situ device
  previous device
Spontaneous
  thoracic outlet syndrome
Medical
  hypercoagulable state
    congenital
    malignancy
      occult
      overt
  low flow
    stasis
      cardiac failure
    external compression
      retrosternal goitre
      aneurysm
      malignancy
  vein injury
    trauma
    drug injection
    post-radiotherapy

Thrombosis associated with temporary or permanent intraluminal devices

Intraluminal diagnostic or therapeutic devices account for 30% of episodes of SAVT. Even in those who have remained asymptomatic, evidence of previous thrombosis is found in up to 40% before a second procedure for vascular access. The incidence of thrombosis is reduced by low-dose anticoagulation (subcutaneous low-dose heparin or mini-dose warfarin).

Spontaneous or effort-related thrombosis

Sometimes termed the *Paget-von Schroetter syndrome*, this is responsible for 30–40% of SAVT and is the outcome of compression as the subclavian vein crosses the first rib to enter the root of the neck and thorax. The vein may be compressed in isolation (10%) or in combination with the subclavian artery or the T1 root of the brachial plexus. Repeated intermittent compression produces damage to the vein wall and results in inflammation with eventual fibrotic stenosis and/or thrombosis. A recent increase in muscle bulk in the shoulder girdle and scalene muscles may also precipitate obstruction.

Other causes

The remaining patients have heterogeneous aetiological factors but can be characterized under one or other of the headings which constitute Virchow's triad (see p. 69): alteration of blood flow; hypercoagulability; and damage to the vessel wall. Low-flow states in severe congestive cardiac failure may be associated with a SAVT. Systemic hypercoagulable states include: deficiency of protein C, protein S, antithrombin III, and lupus inhibitor; the antiphospholipid syndrome; and the presence of anticardiolipin antibodies. Possibly the most common of these will prove to be the recently described abnormalities in factor V which results in resistance to activated protein C. Such conditions, although uncommon, should be suspected in younger patients with a history of thrombotic episodes without obvious precipitating features. Malignant disease (with or without associated radiation fibrosis) accounts for 20% of thromboses and should always be considered in the differential diagnosis even if the initial findings are negative. Extrinsic compression or damage can be the result of: adjacent fractures (clavicle, scapula, first rib or proximal humerus); an anterior dislocation of the humeral head; or, rarely, a congenital abnormality in the insertions of the biceps brachii or latissimus dorsi muscles. Finally, damage to the intima can follow the administration of hypertonic solutions, injection of drugs by addicts in unfavourable circumstances and the inclusion of the subclavian vein in a radiotherapy field.

Other considerations **Pulmonary emboli**
Pulmonary emboli occur in some 2.5% of instances of SAVT and on rare occasions may be of significant size with long-term pulmonary damage and pulmonary hypertension. An implanted device may also be infected and, until it is removed, fungal and opportunistic infections are particularly difficult to diagnose and treat. Septic pulmonary emboli may cause metastatic lung infection.

Side affected In thrombosis which is the result of an indwelling catheter, the left arm is more commonly involved as a consequence of the longer intravenous course of the foreign body and the angulation at the termination of the left brachiocephalic vein. By contrast, in SAVT without obvious precipitating factors, the right arm is affected twice as frequently as the left, probably reflecting the dominance of right handedness in the population.

Physical status In patients whose SAVT is thought to be the result of compression at the thoracic outlet, heavily built males predominate (male to female ratio 3.5:1).

Time of presentation The syndrome may present apparently acutely 24–72 hours following an initiating event such as an injury or a repetitive unusual exercise though there may not be any such history. In catheter-induced lesions, thrombosis may develop clinically some time after the catheter has been removed.

CLINICAL FEATURES The mode of presentation depends, at least in part, on the underlying cause.

Some thromboses, particularly those associated with implants such as catheters, may remain asymptomatic and be discovered only when a further attempt is made to gain access. Typical symptoms of SAVT include aching pain or discomfort in the arm with an associated heaviness, made worse by activity and relieved by rest and elevation. Swelling of the whole arm and stiff fingers associated with non-pitting oedema may extend to the chest wall and be so extensive that the patient complains of swelling of the breast.

On physical examination the arm is usually swollen but the oedema does not pit. The dependent parts of the affected limb may have the mottled, cyanotic appearance of outflow obstruction. Veins are prominent in the hand and forearm and distended collateral superficial veins become evident over the shoulder and anterior chest wall. A palpable, tender thrombosed cord may be present in the basilic or axillary vein. Distension of the ispilateral jugular vein is suggestive of more proximal thrombosis.

Because of the possibility of an underlying malignant process, physical examination must include specific assessment of the breast, pelvis and rectum as well as lymph nodes, especially in the supraclavicular region. Rarely in patients with severe intercurrent medical problems, *phlegmasia cerulea dolens* and *venous gangrene* may complicate the presentation and are often agonal events.

DIAGNOSIS The diagnosis is usually apparent on clinical grounds but should be confirmed by objective tests. Duplex and colour-duplex scanning are highly effective (**Figure 10.1**) and have the advantage of being non-invasive, although scanning in the presence of a catheter is sometimes difficult. Phlebography is used in circumstances where the cause is in some doubt or when duplex scanning is not available. Injection of contrast may often be made via an existing catheter or other prosthetic device such as one that is in use for haemodialysis.

Other non-invasive methods which include infrared scanning or photoplethysmography are not widely used. Their accuracy in the diagnosis of deep venous thrombosis in the lower limbs is less than that of duplex scanning and there is no evidence to suggest that they are any more effective in the arms. CT scanning with contrast and MRI or spiral CT have also been used to diagnose subclavian thrombosis but they are possibly of more value to search for an unsuspected malignancy.

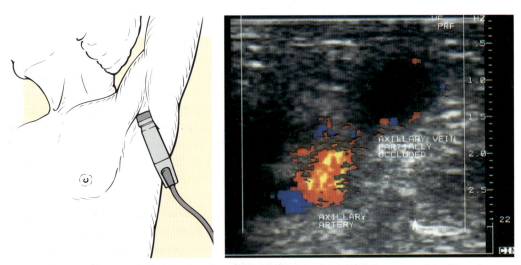

Figure 10.1 Axillary–subclavian vein thrombosis. The thrombosed axillary vein (black) is shown above and to the right of the artery (red). This thrombosis followed shortly after an effort (rapid extension of the arm) in a young ballet dancer.

TREATMENT *Catheter-related thrombosis*

Removal of the catheter and systemic anticoagulation usually relieves symptoms and can lead to resolution of the problem. Should re-cannulation be required, the contralateral side is still usually accessible. However, when extensive or multiple episodes of thrombosis have occurred neither subclavian or jugular vein may be available and the loss of venous access may be critical for the care of the patient. In consequence, delay in removal and extension of the thrombosis may take place in an attempt to preserve the access. Attempted future access may then entail significant additional risk for the patient. However, there are a number of alternatives and individual problems must be discussed in the light of the availability of other routes such as the transfemoral, transiliac and caval via a translumbar approach.

Subclavian vein thrombosis that results from previous or current cannulation may develop proximal to a functioning arteriovenous access. The symptoms are then more severe because of the high inflow pressure; optimum treatment is closure or removal of the fistula. However, venous bypass has been performed with maintenance of access and relief of symptoms.

Thrombosis associated with thoracic outlet syndrome

The diagnosis of thoracic outlet syndrome may not always be clear with many patients presenting with an apparently spontaneous thrombosis. In the absence of identifiable precipitating medical conditions, patients are usually presumed to have a thoracic outlet syndrome. Although the established conservative treatment is anticoagulation with heparin, higher rates of vein patency and reduced rates of long-term symptoms of venous hypertension are said to occur when more aggressive approaches are used. However, prospective randomized trials have not been conducted.

Thrombolytic therapy using urokinase, streptokinase or t-PA have all been demonstrated to be effective in clearing subclavian thrombosis and seem to be more effective than heparin alone. Even higher rates of patency are claimed to result when thrombolysis is combined with surgical decompression of the vein (by first rib excision) and, if required, vein repair (venous patch or balloon venoplasty with or without stenting).

Venous thrombectomy is occasionally performed to relieve venous obstruction and to preserve valvular integrity. However, the operation is seldom successful in that rapid postoperative rethrombosis occurs in most cases if the predisposing extraluminal compression is not removed at the same time. If this can be done long-term patency has been observed after thrombectomy.

Consideration should be always given to relieving the cause of compression to prevent recurrence even if thrombectomy is not used. The site of the most severe compression is usually in the costoclavicular space which should be enlarged by resection of either the clavicle or the first rib by the transaxillary approach.

Thrombosis associated with medical conditions

Treatment is anticoagulation when this is not contraindicated. The nature of the underlying medical condition usually determines outcome. Aggressive management may not be appropriate. However, balloon dilatation and stenting of the subclavian and brachiocephalic veins have been performed for thrombosis caused by malignant external compression.

PROGNOSIS

Rapid recovery from the initial symptoms occurs in most young patients but residual symptoms and signs may occur in some 50–80% of patients treated conservatively. Usually the acute swelling and arm pain disappear within 1–3 weeks. Some patients have persistent or recurrent symptoms such as swelling, numbness, easy fatiguability and episodes of recurrent superficial phlebitis. All symptoms are usually made worse by exercise.

It has been observed in some reports that the incidence of late symptoms may be reduced by effective, early thrombectomy.

BIBLIOGRAPHY

Ameli FM *et al.* Consequences of 'conservative' conventional management of axillary vein thrombosis. *Can J Surg* 1987; **30**: 167.

Bern MM, Lokich JJ, Wallach SR. Very low doses of warfarin can prevent thrombosis in central venous catheters. A randomized prospective trial. *Ann Intern Med* 1990; **112**: 423.

Bonnet F, Loriferne JF, Texier JP *et al.* Evaluation of Doppler examination for diagnosis of catheter-related deep vein thrombosis. *Intens Care Med* 1989; **15**: 238.

Brochner G, Rojas M, Armas AJ *et al.* Axillary-subclavian venous thrombosis. *J Cardiovasc Surg* 1989; **30**: 108.

Chandrasekhar R, Nott DM, Enabi L *et al.* Upper limb venous gangrene, a lethal condition. *Eur J Vasc Surg* 1993; **7**: 475.

Fabri PJ *et al.* Incidence and prevention of thrombosis of the subclavian vein during total parenteral nutrition. *Surg Gynecol Obstet* 1982; **155**: 238.

Freund HR. Chemical phlebothrombosis of large veins: a not uncommon complication of total parenteral nutrition. *Arch Surg* 1981; **116**: 1220.

Gould JR, Carloss HW, Skinner WL. Groshong catheter-associated subclavian vein thrombosis. *Am J Med* 1993; **95**: 419.

Hardman D, Englund R, Hanel K. Aspects of central venous catheter usage in patients with malignancy. *N Z Med J* 1994; **197**: 186.

Kerr TM, Lutter KS, Moeller DM *et al.* Upper extremity venous thrombosis diagnosed by duplex scanning. *Am J Surg* 1990; **160**: 202.

Kraybill WG, Allen BT. Preoperative duplex venous imaging in the assessment of patients with venous access. *J Surg Oncol* 1993; **52**: 244.

Machleder HL. Evaluation of a new treatment for Paget–Schroetter syndrome: spontaneous thrombosis of the axillary-subclavian vein. *J Vasc Surg* 1993; **17**: 305.

Nemmers DW, Thorpe PE, Knibbe MA *et al.* Upper extremity venous thrombosis. Case report and literature review. *Orthop Rev* 1990; **19**: 164.

Sanders RJ, Haug C. Subclavian vein obstruction and thoracic outlet syndrome: a review of etiology and management. *Ann Vasc Surg* 1990; **4**: 397.

Thompson RM, Schneider PA, Nelken NA *et al.* Circumferential venolysis and paraclavicular thoracic outlet decompression for 'effort thrombosis' of the subclavian vein. *J Vasc Surg* 1992; **32**: 723.

Chronic venous insufficiency and postphlebitic syndrome

GENERAL CONSIDERATIONS

The principal late complication of deep vein thrombosis is chronic venous insufficiency (CVI). Most patients with serious problems have originally had an iliofemoral thrombosis and between 20 and 87% give a history of such an episode; in others it may have been asymptomatic. Follow-up of patients after a documented episode of deep vein thrombosis reveals that up to 86% may be expected to develop a venous ulcer within 10 years. However, as long as 15 years may elapse before CVI appears. Persistent obstruction from incomplete recanalization of the thrombosed veins, destruction of deep valves and reflux through incompetent perforator veins all cause high pressure in the superficial venous system.

CVI is widespread, serious and often underestimated in terms of its clinical and social importance. It affects some 0.5% of the populations of the UK and USA. Female patients are twice as common as males. The mean age of presentation for females is 55 and 10% are hospitalized at least once because of recurrent thrombosis, cellulitis, lipodermatosclerosis and venous ulceration or for surgical treatment. It has been calculated that two million workdays are lost in the USA each year because of complications caused by CVI.

In that the majority of cases are probably the late aftermath of deep venous thrombosis, the term *postphlebitic syndrome* is generally used as a synonym for CVI. However, this is not necessarily appropriate in that other factors (congenital absence or incompetence of the valves, congenital or chronic dilatation of the deep venous system) may initiate CVI. Ferris and Kistner in 1982 identified a population with primary incompetence of the valves of deep veins. It may be that some patients thought to have had a silent deep venous thrombosis suffer instead from this syndrome. It is further possible that the incompetent valves may themselves be associated with a higher incidence of deep venous thrombosis.

The exact structural cause in an individual patient with CVI may not be identified when non-operative medical management is successful. However, when direct reconstruction of the deep venous system is planned—as discussed on p. 136—surgery must be planned on the basis of a clear understanding of the particular disease process and of its anatomy.

The acute onset in a previously healthy patient (particularly an elderly one) of deep venous insufficiency associated with signs of obstruction suggest the need to search for any of the extrinsic causes of compression considered in Chapter 6.

PATHOPHYSIOLOGY

The development of the sequelae of a deep venous thrombosis is still unclear and confusing. In the months that follow the event, recanalization of the veins restores patency but competence of the valves is often lost. Valves distal to the thrombus are thought to dilate sequentially as the proximal incompetent venous segment transmits an abnormally high hydrostatic pressure to the next distal valve. The increase in venous pressure is eventually transmitted to the perforating veins which dilate with loss of competence and temporary reversal of venous flow with changes in posture.

The importance of the combination of progressive deep and perforating venous valvular incompetence has been emphasized by Yao and his colleagues. Incompetent valves in perforating veins are, however, the commonest finding in CVI and in one study were present in 60% of patients as compared with 27% who had incompetent valves in deep veins. Nevertheless the presence of deep venous valvular incompetence correlates well with symptomatic chronic venous insufficiency. Perhaps the best objective correlate of symptomatic CVI is popliteal valve incompetence.

Increased pressure in the deep veins as a consequence of incompetent valves is transmitted through incompetent perforators to the venous end of the capillary loop. In consequence the architecture of the microcirculation is altered and changes take place in the skin and subcutaneous tissues. An increased exchange surface is the result of elongation and dilatation of the capillaries which take on a glomerular-like appearance with thickening of the capillary wall (**Figures 11.1** and **11.2**).

Figure 11.1
Massive dilatation of venules and capillaries in the subcutaneous tissue in a limb with venous hypertensive microangiopathy distally to a venous ulcer (section from the medial perimalleolar region).

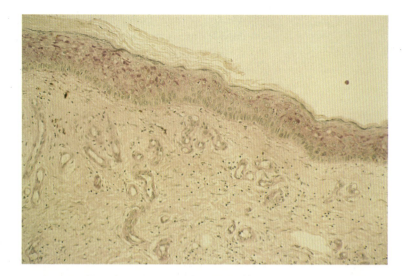

Figure 11.2
The dilatation and glomerular-like aspect of the capillaries which increases the exchange surface and the thickening of the capillary wall is evident in this section.

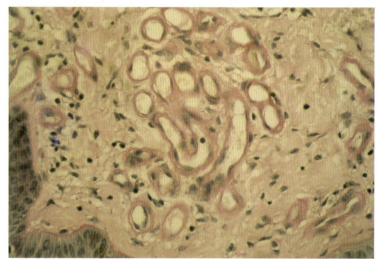

In association with these changes, there is an increase in capillary filtration. The increased venular hydrostatic pressure reduces reabsorption of fluid and protein from the interstitial space with resulting oedema which is often the first clinical manifestation of CVI. Venous oedema initially appears in the evening, involving the ankle and lower leg, and recedes at night. It may progress with time so that the leg eventually does not return to normal after a night's rest and the swelling includes progressively more of the leg up to and beyond the knee. Massive swelling of the entire extremity or of both legs may be seen with iliac or inferior vena cava occlusion.

Congestion and cyanosis of the skin imply capillary hypoxia and this can lead to diapedesis of red cells which disintegrate in the interstitial space to deposit haemosiderin and cause brown pigmentation. A further pathophysiological change that has been postulated is an increased escape of fibrin through the capillary wall. The presence of this and of its degradation products leads to a dense, pericapillary 'cuff' which cannot be cleared by normal fibrinolysis—which may also be locally impaired in CVI. The cuff is thought to act as a barrier to the diffusion of gas, nutrients and metabolites, so interfering with the nutrition of the subcutaneous tissues and predisposing to ischaemia and necrosis. However, the concept has been challenged and remains unconfirmed. The best that can be said at the moment is that multiple factors appear to be in action in determining the microcirculatory changes observed in venous hypertension and more research is needed in this field.

Some research suggests that in CVI skin oxygen tensions are decreased but this has not always been confirmed. The possible effects of an increase in skin PCO_2 in promoting and maintaining local vasodilatation is still not fully understood.

CLINICAL FEATURES   Many of these are apparent from the pathophysiological changes that have been described. The initial symptoms may be confined to nocturnal swelling which is usually progressive and eventually becomes irreversible. Pain is not a usual feature until ulceration occurs but some patients complain of pain in the muscles of the leg after prolonged standing; resting supine or elevating the leg generally relieves aching and fatigue. CVI associated with long-standing severe iliofemoral–femoral obstruction and a patent distal venous system may give rise to *venous claudication*—a severe, bursting pain, usually in the calf on walking. The pain is the result of venous congestion, made worse with exercise because the increased arterial and venous flow associated with muscle activity cannot be returned to the heart as fast as it is delivered, particularly if there is a poor collateral circulation. The pain of venous claudication is probably secondary to a further rise in pressure within the musculofascial compartments which are known to have an increased resting pressure and water content in iliofemoral thrombosis. Dermatitis causes itching and may make the patient scratch and precipitate an ulcer. Ulceration caused by CVI is slow to heal and generally recurs if the underlying cause of venous hypertension is not corrected.

The appearances on clinical examination vary with the extent to which the disorder has advanced. There may only be swelling or this may be accompanied by any or all of the more obvious features—secondary varicosities, skin pigmentation and cyanosis, eczema, dermatitis and ulceration.

DIAGNOSIS   The clinical diagnosis is usually easily made on history and physical examination. The differential diagnoses include other causes of dependent oedema such as congestive heart failure or chronic renal disease and lymphoedema. Differentiating CVI from the latter occasionally causes difficulty. Lymphoedema involves the limb in a uniform way, the subcutaneous tissues are usually firmer than in venous disease and there is rarely pitting.

Ulceration can be the result of a combination of arterial and venous disease (**Table 11.1**). Painful skin lesions located distally in the foot or toes, skin pallor and diminished or absent arterial pulsation are features of arterial involvement. If oedema or chronic thickening of the skin makes clinical examination of the pulses difficult, non-invasive arterial studies in the vascular laboratory should be undertaken.

Table 11.1
Classification of leg ulceration

Vascular	Systemic and metabolic
Arterial	Ulcerative colitis
Atherosclerosis	Diabetes
Arteriovenous fistula	Sickle cell anaemia
Thromboangiitis obliterans	Avitaminosis
Polyarteritis nodosa	
Hypertension	**Neoplastic**
Vasospastic disease – Raynaud's	Primary skin tumours
	Kaposi sarcoma
Venous	melanoma
Chronic venous insufficiency	squamous cell carcinoma
deep valvular incompetence or	leukaemia
deep to superficial valvular	metastatic tumours
incompetence	
misplaced sclerotherapy or	**Traumatic**
drug injection	Radiation
	Thermal burn
Lymphatic	Pressure necrosis
Lymphoedema	Insect bites
Infective	**Neurotrophic**
Chronic osteomyelitis, either	Cord lesions
primary or secondary to fracture	Peripheral neuropathies
Pyogenic	trauma
Synergistic gangrene (Meleney's	diabetes
ulcer)	tabes dorsalis
Other rare causes	alcoholism
syphilis	
tuberculosis	
leishmaniasis	
leprosy	
fungal disease	

LOCALIZATION AND QUANTIFICATION

General

Though physical examination usually reveals the presence of CVI, it is not sufficiently precise to localize and quantify the underlying anatomical and functional defects.

In some limbs incompetence of the deep valves may be localized to either femoral or popliteal veins, causing venous hypertension in a venous segment. Alternatively, the valvular incompetence may be generalized. As has been mentioned, valvular incompetence in the popliteal vein is believed to correlate most directly with the classical features of CVI, particularly ulceration, although femoral incompetence is the most important causal factor and some 5% of patients have proximal incompetence either localized or in conjunction with distal incompetence.

If there is no apparent venous thrombosis or deep venous valvular insufficiency, other possibilities must be evaluated. Pelvic tumours, haemangiomas and arteriovenous fistulas may give rise to chronic, rapidly progressive, venous insufficiency as may primary valvular agenesis.

Phlebography

Of the two techniques, *ascending* and *descending*, the former has been for many years the standard with which new diagnostic tests are compared. The patency of deep veins and of perforators can be easily demonstrated as well as postphlebitic changes and chronic obstruction. Ascending phlebography can define valvular incompetence by inducing a rise in venous pressure with a Valsalva manoeuvre.

If reconstructive surgery for the deep system is under consideration, a clear definition of the state of the venous valves usually requires descending phlebography. The technique is a fluoroscopic, dynamic study and provides functional as well as anatomical information; however, it is considered by some to be of uncertain value

Table 11.2 Interpretation of descending phlebography

Complete competence
No retrograde flow during full Valsalva manoeuvre

Satisfactory competence
Mild leakage limited to the thigh during full Valsalva manoeuvre

Moderate incompetence
Prominent leakage into calf during Valsalva manoeuvre
Prograde flow maintained in iliac vein

Severe incompetence
Cascading retrograde flow during Valsalva manoeuvre
Reflux into calf perforators

because of differences in technique and interpretation. A grading system has been developed by Kistner to evaluate descending phlebography (**Table 11.2**). Decisions on valvular replacement or reconstruction are dependent on the results of such anatomical and functional assessment.

The roles of ambulatory venous pressure (AVP) measurements and other non-invasive and invasive tests are described in Chapter 4. They allow definition of the structural nature of the problem, quantitation of the degree of venous hypertension and the study over time of the development of the disorder and the effects of intervention.

NON-OPERATIVE TREATMENT

Medical management remains the most common form of treatment for the majority of patients with CVI. Education of patients to understand the chronic and insidious nature of their problem is a difficult but essential basis of continued care. Many physicians fail to understand the slow, progressive evolution of CVI and often their patients do not appreciate the necessity for prolonged therapy.

The most important aim of therapy is to control venous hypertension and avoid oedema. This may be achieved in most patients with graduated elastic stockings. However, when there is a bone or joint problem or any other cause of restricted mobility, even elastic compression may be disappointing in its effects and enforced active or formal passive movement may be crucial to assure improvement. Intermittent periods of leg elevation and avoidance of prolonged sitting and standing should be advised. Knee-length stockings are usually sufficient because most of the muscular action which promotes venous return is in the calf, the highest venous pressure is below the knee and in consequence complications of venous insufficiency are practically never seen above this level.

Unless the venous problem can be dealt with, either by control of deep to superficial incompetence or by reconstruction of deep valves, elastic support is often a lifelong necessity. Strict adherence to the use of stockings often prevents the consequences of chronic venous hypertension and may alleviate symptoms and prevent the progression of changes in the skin and subcutaneous tissues. Stockings which produce 30–40 mmHg compression at the level of the ankle are generally very effective in reducing oedema and other signs of venous insufficiency. Heavier stockings are advisable for patients with associated lymphoedema or refractory venous oedema.

Ulceration is often treated conservatively with elevation, medication and compressive therapy, usually on an outpatient basis. Semi-rigid zinc oxide bandages (Unna's boots) are still used extensively and, provided that the technique is rigorous, can be successful in healing an ulcer. The immobilization of the ankle joint with this treatment method is possible and should be prevented by using the bandage for not more than 2 to 3 weeks.

Antibiotics or antibacterial solutions are indicated only in patients with documented bacterial contamination. If cellulitis supervenes, the most appropriate antibiotics are used either locally or systemically after identifying the predominant organism present.

Allergies to local treatment must be noted and prevented because local allergic reactions can turn small ulcerations into larger skin defects which are more difficult to heal. Eczema and dermatitis are treated when appropriate with lanolin solutions, aluminium subacetate, steroid preparations or antibiotics.

Extensive ulceration with associated cellulitis may require hospitalization and elevation of the leg. Skin grafting may be needed in some patients. Large, recurrent ulcerations are an indication for more aggressive management.

SURGICAL MANAGEMENT

Superficial incompetence

In patients who have superficial valvular incompetence at the saphenofemoral junction and/or elsewhere but a normal deep system, interruption of the sites of incompetence and sclerotherapy for residual superficial varices corrects venous hypertension in the superficial system. This may be achieved by selective surgery after identification (by colour-duplex or phlebography) of all incompetent venous sites. Often this type of surgery may be performed on an outpatient basis in repeated short sessions. Sclerotherapy of the more proximal incompetent veins appears to be less effective than that for veins below the knee. Often one or two perforators may be identified close to an ulcer. Ligation and sclerotherapy of these is useful to decrease local venous hypertension to a level associated with more rapid healing.

More systematic operations, such as extrafascial or subfascial ligations which interrupt incompetent perforators, may still have a place when multiple incompetent communicating veins (documented and localized by phlebography or non-invasive tests) are the major problem. Extensive dissection can now be avoided as it is possible to use colour-duplex precisely to localize incompetent perforators (**Figure 11.3**).

Figure 11.3
The localization of incompetent perforators causing or increasing venous hypertension (a) is now easy and possible with duplex and colour-duplex. (b) The superficial incompetent vein, the perforating vein and the deep system (posterior tibial vein, below) are shown in the same section.

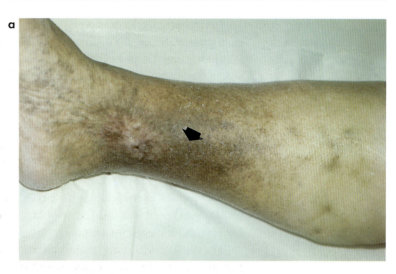

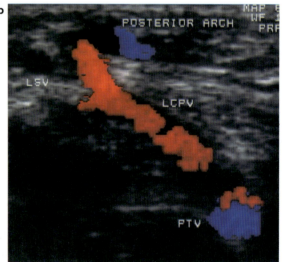

Even when both deep and superficial systems are involved, the correction of superficial venous hypertension may often be followed by a very relevant clinical result (for example, healing of an ulcer). Contrary to what has been taught in the past, removal of secondary varicosities in the saphenous systems does not, except in rare instances, impair venous return from the extremity.

Supplementary surgery for intractable ulcer

If an ulcer cannot be controlled by conservative management or surgery to the superficial system or if it is very large, local surgery is indicated. Split-thickness skin grafts may be applied directly to a clean granulating ulcer or the ulcer may be excised and a skin graft applied primarily. However, recurrences are common if nothing is done to correct the venous disorder.

Valvular incompetence in the deep system

The long-term results of direct surgical correction of deep insufficiency are still being evaluated. In consequence, such procedures should be undertaken in well defined clinical circumstances and by specialized centres only. The important role of coexistent incompetent valves in perforating veins in aggravating CVI may be overlooked and in such circumstances re-establishment of competence in the deep venous system will fail. Incompetent perforators should be treated at the time of deep venous reconstruction.

Newer procedures have been and are being developed on the basis of a better understanding of venous pathophysiology. However, controversy remains over the importance of creating a single, competent valve at the level of the superficial femoral vein and the importance of femoral versus popliteal incompetence. Assessment of such issues is difficult because it is necessary to follow up patients for many years after reconstruction.

Finally, the use of surgical rather than medical treatment must rest on a satisfactory though difficult cost–benefit analysis of both.

Surgery for CVI which is the outcome of a deep venous disorder may be divided into two main categories:

♦ operations to restore patency;
♦ operations to restore venous competence.

Patency

Operations to restore patency are applicable to only a small minority of patients with CVI because only 8% with the condition have significant obstruction. At present there are three types of operations:

♦ the Husni operation;
♦ the Palma–Dale operation and its variants;
♦ direct reconstructions of the iliac vein and the inferior vena cava.

The *Husni operation or in situ saphenopopliteal veno-venous bypass* aims to relieve obstruction of the femoral and popliteal veins by using the ipsilateral saphenous vein anastomosed end-to-side to the most proximal patent deep vein, usually the popliteal (**Figure 11.4**). Free vein grafts can be used if the ipsilateral saphenous vein is not suitable and provided the other extremity is not involved.

In the *Palma–Dale operation* iliac obstruction is bypassed with the contralateral saphenous vein (**Figure 11.5**). The best results are obtained when the procedure is used to relieve extrinsic compression in which the veins themselves are structurally intact. In consequence, patients treated by this procedure have often been those

Figure 11.4 The Husni operation (see text).

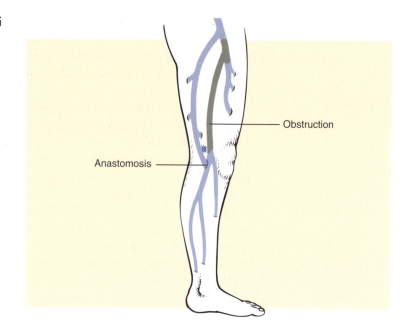

Figure 11.5 The Palma–Dale operation to bypass deep venous (iliac) obstruction.

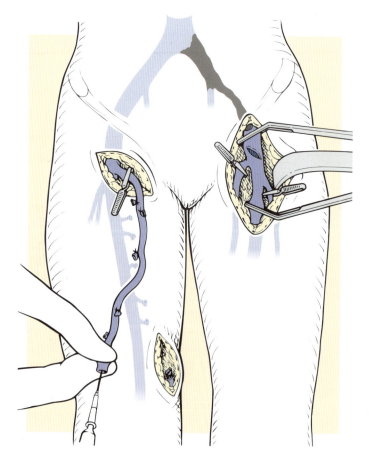

with malignant obstruction of the iliac vein (43% overall and 65% of those over 50). A further urgent indication is to prevent the development of venous gangrene. In such circumstances, outflow is generally good as the venous system contralateral to the obstruction is normal.

Unless there is an acute obstruction which requires urgent treatment, dynamic tests should be undertaken before surgery to indicate clearly the site and nature of an outflow obstruction. If patency of collaterals is such that distal venous pressures, even after exercise, are only mildly elevated, bypass grafting cannot be expected to be successful.

In the *Palma procedure* an alternative to the saphenous vein is an externally reinforced PTFE graft. Arteriovenous fistulas are often created at the time of operation to increase flow rates through the graft in the first postoperative days. They are usually temporary and ligated or occluded after 6–12 weeks.

Direct reconstructions of the iliac veins and the superior and inferior vena cavae have been performed with spiral vein grafts

Figure 11.5 (continued)

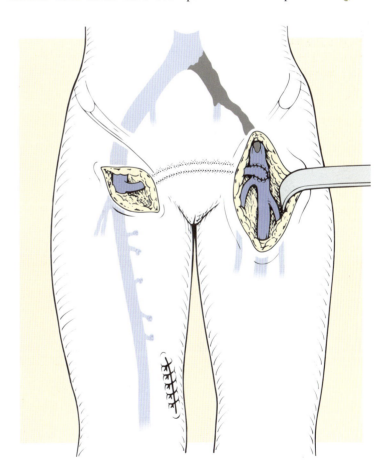

and with externally supported (ringed) PTFE grafts. Results are promising and it may be that direct reconstructions will prove better than extra-anatomical operations. Temporary arteriovenous fistulas and anticoagulation as adjuvant therapy are recommended with these procedures.

Restoration of competence

There are a number of operations. They include external vein valvuloplasty, transplants of valve-containing segments of brachial vein to the femoral or popliteal levels, and vein-segment transpositions.

External valvuloplasty can be performed after demonstrating the presence of mobile valvular cusps in the vein by high resolution duplex scanning or phlebography. After careful 'no-touch' dissection of the vein, the valvular structure is isolated (**Figure 11.6**) and the valvular ring is made smaller by two opposite, continuous

Figure 11.6 Careful dissection of the superficial femoral vein allows the valve cusps to be seen through the vein wall.

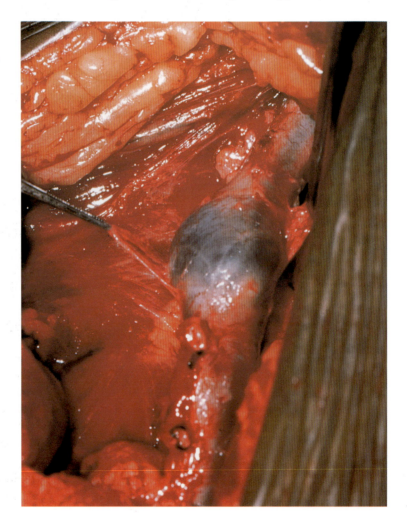

Figure 11.7 Steps of external valvuloplasty (Kistner) to reduce the diameter of the valvular ring at the cusps so making the venous segment competent.

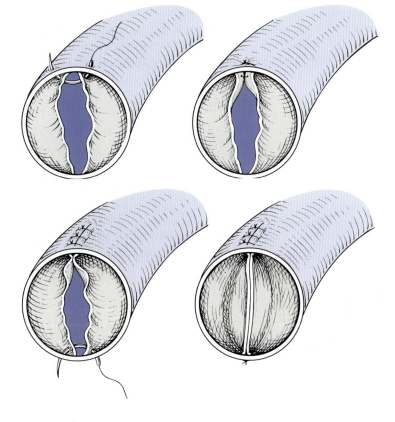

Figure 11.8 The modified procedure of anterior plication limits vein dissection.

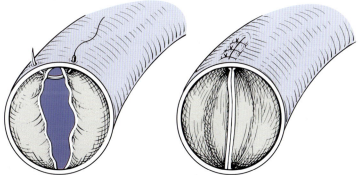

sutures (1–2 cm) along the commissures of the cusps (**Figure 11.7**). Valvuloplasty gives good results when the incompetence is mainly the outcome of dilatation of the vein and the cusps are functionally intact. Some dilatation of the venous segment is often observed months after valvuloplasty and reinforcements of the venous walls around the corrected valvular ring—nets, venous cuffs—have been recommended. Recently a different type of *limited anterior valvuloplasty* including only the anterior surface of the valvular ring has been developed (**Figure 11.8**). This is often effec-

Figure 11.9 Significant reflux in an incompetent superficial femoral vein demonstrated by duplex.

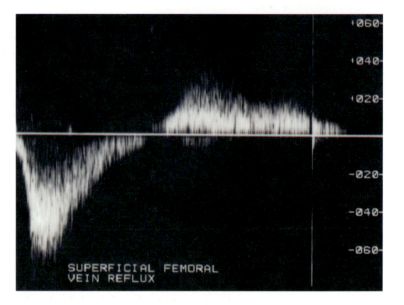

tive in making the femoral vein competent: the limited dissection preserves both the vasa vasorum and innervation and is not followed by dilatation of the vein. **Figure 11.9** shows incompetence of the superficial femoral vein (associated in this case with incompetence of the popliteal and more distal veins)—an indication for valvuloplasty.

External valvuloplasty has recently been performed with angioscopy to control the approximation of the vein cusps (*Glowinski–Merrell–Bower method*).

That valvuloplasty is effective in restoring competence can be confirmed by B-mode ultrasound imaging during a Valsalva manoeuvre when correct approximation and superimposition of the valve cusps is demonstrated (**Figure 11.10**).

Figure 11.10 The echogenic (white) line formed by the two cusps superimposed during a Valsalva manoeuvre after valvuloplasty of the vein as shown in Figure 11.8. The echogenic line was not visible before valvuloplasty.

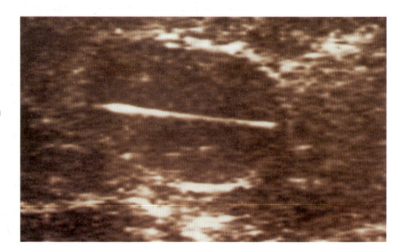

The results of valvuloplasty in highly specialized centres are satisfactory but patient selection and surgical techniques are still controversial. The majority of patients are probably best managed nonoperatively. The 14-year results reported by Ferris and Kistner in 1982 are encouraging and these difficult venous reconstructions may be performed in selected subjects when medical management is unsatisfactory. Though at this moment the techniques of investigation and surgical methods make valvuloplasty practical, more and larger long-term prospective studies are needed to confirm its efficacy and the best indications.

COMPLICATIONS AND PROGNOSIS

Rarely, after many years, a chronic ulcer may undergo malignant transformation (Marjolin's ulcer), a change that is not always easy to recognize. Therefore, intractable ulcers should undergo biopsy.

Recurrent phlebitis and thrombosis are more frequent than previously believed and may produce a progressive deterioration of the venous system. To avoid this complication requires prophylactic measures such as elastic support, periodic elevation of the legs and avoidance of trauma and situations that promote venous hypertension.

BIBLIOGRAPHY

Belcaro G. Femoral vein valve repair with limited anterior plication (LAP). *J Cardiovasc Surg* 1993; **34**: 77.

Belcaro G, Christopoulos D, Nicolaides AN. Venous insufficiency: noninvasive testing. In: Bergan J, Kistner R, eds. *Atlas of Venous Surgery*. Philadelphia: Saunders, 1992; 9–24.

Belcaro G, Labropoulos N, Christopoulos D *et al*. Non-invasive test in venous insufficiency. *J Cardiovasc Surg* 1993; **34**: 3.

Belcaro G, Nicolaides AN. Laser-Doppler, oxygen and CO_2 tension in venous hypertension. In: Bernstein EF, ed. *Vascular Diagnosis*. 4th ed. St Louis: Mosby-Year Book, Inc., 1993; 934.

Belcaro G, Rulo A, *et al*. Combined evaluation of postphlebitic limbs by laser-Doppler flowmetry and transcutaneous PO_2/PCO_2 measurements. *Vasa* 1988; **17**: 259.

Bernstein EF, ed. *Vascular Diagnosis*. 4th ed. St Louis: Mosby-Year Book, Inc., 1993.

Browse NL, Burnand KG. The postphlebitic syndrome: a new look. In: Bergan JJ, Yao JST. *Venous Problems*. Chicago: Year Book Medical Publishers, 1978, 395.

Browse NL, Gray L, *et al*. Blood and vein wall fibrinolytic activity in health and vascular disease. *Br Med J* 1977; **1**: 478.

Christopoulos D, Nicolaides AN. Noninvasive diagnosis and quantitation of popliteal reflux in the swollen and ulcerated leg. *J Cardiovasc Surg* 1988; **29**: 535.

Christopoulos D, Nicolaides AN, Cook A *et al*. Pathogenesis of venous ulceration in relation to the calf muscle pump function. *Surgery* 1989; **106**: 829.

Christopoulos DC, Nicolaides AN, Belcaro G *et al*. Venous hypertensive microangiopathy in relation to clinical severity and effect of elastic compression. *J Dermatol Surg Oncol* 1991; **17**: 809.

Dale WA. Crossover grafts for iliofemoral venous occlusion. In: Bergan JJ, Yao JST, eds. *Venous Problems*. Chicago: Year Book Medical Publishers, 1978: 411.

Dale WA, Harris J, Terry RB. Polytetrafluoroethylene reconstruction of the inferior vena cava. *Surgery* 1984; **95**: 625.

Dodd H, Cockett FB. *The Pathology and Surgery of the Veins of the Lower Limb*. Edinburgh & London: Churchill Livingstone, 1976.

Dodd HJ, Gaylarde PM, Sarkany I. Skin oxygen tension in venous insufficiency of the lower leg. *J R Soc Med* 1985; **78**: 373.

Dollmar JF, Hutschenreiter S. Vascular prostheses for the venous system. In: Chan EL, Bardin JA, Bernstein EF. Inferior vena cava bypass: experimental evaluation of externally supported grafts and initial clinical application. *J Vasc Surg* 1984; **1**: 675.

Ferris EB, Kistner RL. Femoral vein reconstruction in the management of chronic venous insufficiency. *Arch Surg* 1982; **117**: 1571.

Franzeck UK, Bollinger A, *et al*. Transcutaneous oxygen tension and capillary morphologic characteristics and density in patients with chronic venous incompetence. *Circulation* 1984; **70**: 806.

Glowinski P, Merrell SW, Bower TC. Femoral vein valve repair under direct vision without venotomy: a modified technique with angioscopy. *J Vasc Surg* 1992; **14**: 645.

Gloviczki P, Hollier LH, *et al*. Experimental replacement of the inferior vena cava: factors affecting patency. *Surgery* 1984; **6**: 657.

Goldstone, J. Veins and Lymphatics. In: Way LW, ed. *Current Surgical Diagnosis and Treatment*. 10th ed., East Norwalk,USA: Appleton and Lange, 1994; 78.

Husni EA. Clinical experience with femoropopliteal venous reconstruction. In: Bergan JJ, Yao JST, eds. *Venous Problems*. Chicago: Year Book Medical Publishers, 1978: 485.

Johnson ND, Queral LA, *et al*. Late objective assessment of venous valve surgery. *Arch Surg* 1981; **116**: 1461.

Kistner RL. Diagnosis of chronic venous insufficiency. *J Vasc Surg* 1986; **3**: 185.

Kohler TR, Strandness DE Jr. Noninvasive testing for the evaluation of chronic venous disease. *World J Surg* 1986; **10**: 903.

Laurora G, Pizzicannella G, *et al*. Skin flux and histology in venous hypertension. *Vasc Surg* 1993; **27**: 110.

Nachbur B. Assessment of venous disorders by venous pressure measurements. In: Hobbs JT, ed. *The Treatment of Venous Disorders.* Philadelphia: JB Lippincott Co, 1977.

Nicolaides AN, Hoare M, Miles CR *et al*. Value of ambulatory venous pressure in the assessment of venous insufficiency. *Vasc Diagn Ther* 1981; **3**: 41.

Nicolaides AN, Zukowski AJ. The value of dynamic venous pressure measurements. *World J Surg* 1986; **10**: 919.

Palma EC, Esperon R. Vein transplants and grafts in the surgical treatment of the postphlebitic syndrome. *J Cardiovasc Surg* 1960; **1**: 94.

Plate G, Brudin L, *et al*. Physiologic and therapeutic aspects in congenital vein valve aplasia of the lower limb. *Ann Surg* 1983; **198**: 299.

Queral LA, Whitehouse WM Jr, *et al*. Surgical correction of chronic deep venous insufficiency by valvular transposition. *Surgery* 1980; **87**: 688.

Qvarfordt P, Eklof B, *et al*. Intramuscular pressure, blood flow, and skeletal muscle metabolism in patients with venous claudication. *Surgery* 1984; **95**: 191.

Raju S. Venous insufficiency of the lower limb and stasis ulceration: changing concepts in management. *Ann Surg* 1983; **197**: 688.

Raju S. New approaches to the diagnosis and treatment of venous obstruction. *J Vasc Surg* 1986; **4(1)**: 42.

Shull KC, Nicolaides AN, *et al*. Significance of popliteal reflux in relation to ambulatory venous pressure and ulceration. *Arch Surg* 1979; **114**: 1304.

Szendro G, Nicolaides AN, *et al*. Duplex scanning in the assessment of deep venous incompetence. *J Vasc Surg* 1986; **4**: 237.

Taheri SA, Pendergast DR, *et al*. Vein valve transplantation. *Am J Surg* 1985; **150**: 201.

Taheri SA, Pendergast D, *et al*. Continuous ambulatory venous pressure for diagnosis of venous insufficiency. Preliminary report. *Am J Surg* 1985; **150**: 203.

Vasdekis SN, Clarke H, Nicolaides AN. Quantification of venous reflux by means of duplex scanning. *J Vasc Surg* 1989; **10**: 670.

Yao JST, Flinn WR, *et al*. The role of noninvasive testing in the evaluation of chronic venous problems. *World J Surg* 1986; **10**: 911.

CHAPTER 12

The swollen limb

**GENERAL
CONSIDERATIONS**

Swelling and oedema are a consequence of an increased production and/or decreased removal of interstitial fluid. An imbalance develops between the filtration pressure in the proximal capillary and the combination of absorptive osmotic and hydrostatic pressure at the venous end. The glomerular-like appearance of capillaries in chronic venous insufficiency and the associated increase in the exchange surface (Figures 11.1 and 11.2, Chapter 11) contribute to this imbalance with accumulation of water and proteins in the interstitial fluid. Large protein molecules, which filter in small quantities through the capillary membrane, are returned to the systemic circulation via the distal lymphatic system which is the most important drainage route from the interstitial space for particulate matter. Decrease in the rate of removal of interstitial proteins is the most important abnormality in lymphoedema. In addition, in chronic venous insufficiency, compression of the distal lymphatic branches because of oedema reduces their drainage capacity. Proteins in the interstitial space increase oncotic pressure which promotes water retention that may become clinically evident as oedema.

The most common causes of limb oedema are indicated in **Table 12.1**.

Primary venous or lymphatic problems, systemic or external causes (e.g. compression by tumours) are associated with acute or chronic oedema of the limbs. In the lower limbs the problem is aggravated by gravity (standing) and partially or completely relieved by elevation.

Table 12.1 Clinical problems causing limb swelling

Systemic causes
Congestive heart failure
Hormone/drug treatment (e.g. some calcium antagonists)
Nephrosis
Cirrhosis
Myxoedema
Hypoproteinaemia

Venous
Chronic venous insufficiency
Extrinsic compression (tumours, retroperitoneal fibrosis, compression by the iliac artery on the left iliac vein)
Arteriovenous communications (AV fistulas)
Trauma (surgery, ligation of veins, caval plication, clipping)

Lymphatic
Primary lymphoedema
    congenital lymphoedema
    early lymphoedema
    late lymphoedema
Secondary lymphoedema
    filariasis
    infections
    neoplastic disease
    radiation
Injury, insect bites, surgical excision of lymph nodes (e.g. mastectomy)
Limb inactivity (e.g. paralysis)

In *acute venous obstruction* oedema is the result of the increased pressure at the venular end of the capillary and reduced reabsorption of fluid. As already mentioned, the interstitial pressure increase because of oedema also excludes by compression some of the terminal lymphatics, further impairing local drainage.

In *chronic venous insufficiency (CVI)*, oedema is mainly the consequence of the persistence of venous hypertension. Most lymphatics still remove extracellular protein and in consequence fluid in chronic venous oedema is low in protein.

The clinical presence of oedema always indicates that the formation of interstitial fluid and lymph exceed resorption. Whatever the cause, chronic oedema produces comparable patterns of secondary inflammation and fibrosis because of the presence of proteins in the interstitial space. If the swelling is unilateral, the causative disorder is generally local (e.g. postmastectomy oedema) and the most frequent diagnostic problem is to decide whether the origin is venous or lymphatic. The presence of external compression from tumours or a history of previous surgery involving lymph nodes may be relevant. In bilateral oedema, systemic causes of swelling (e.g. cardiac) must be excluded.

Occasionally unilateral atrophy of the muscles of one leg (usually in the calf) may confuse the clinical picture by suggesting that there is swelling of the contralateral limb. Also, relative venous hypertension because of decreased mobility (e.g. following paralysis) of a limb is often associated with oedema in the absence of a venous or lymphatic problem.

The presence of swelling is based in most instances on the clinical findings. However, investigations of the venous and lymphatic systems (duplex and colour-duplex, venography or lymphangiography) can be very useful.

Sudden unexplained swelling of the lower limb, particularly in an elderly patient, suggests the presence of extrinsic compression of the great veins within the abdomen. A chest radiograph and imaging of the abdomen by ultrasound and an abdominal CT scan are often indicated.

Treatment depends on the cause. Unilateral oedema from venous or lymphatic problems may generally be controlled with elastic compression and leg elevation. When physical measures are not effective, other possibilities (e.g. surgery aimed to eliminate compression or to restore patency of the deep venous system) should be considered but is the province of specialized units.

VENOUS CONDITIONS LEADING TO A SWOLLEN LIMB

Deep venous thrombosis and chronic venous insufficiency

These common causes of limb swelling are considered in Chapters 6 and 11.

Arterial compression of the common iliac vein

One special problem is unilateral swelling of the distal leg and foot—usually the left—in the presence of an apparently normal venous system and without any other obvious cause. The veins are patent on ultrasound examination, flow is phasic with respiration and is augmented by manual compression of the calf. In such circumstances it is possible that a partial compression of the left common iliac vein by the right common iliac artery may be the cause.

The condition is the outcome of an exaggeration of the normal anatomy of the right common iliac artery and the left common iliac vein. Particularly in young women, the latter is displaced forwards

Figure 12.1 Types of iliac vein compression by the proximal right iliac artery. The compression (with the section of the vein indicated) may range from a partial one which does not affect flow (a) to total occlusion (d).

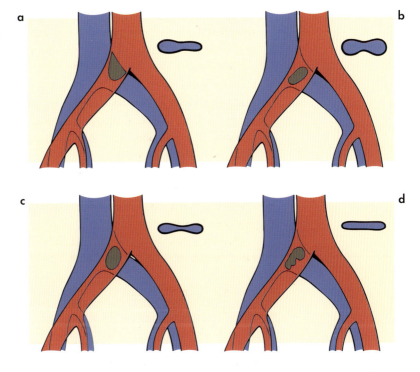

against the relatively unyielding artery by the convexity of the lower lumbar vertebrae. A degree of compression over the termination of the left common iliac vein then results (**Figure 12.1**). On iliac phlebography a filling defect at this site may be observed in half of normal subjects (**Figure 12.1**). The compression is usually compensated for by an increase in the side-to-side cross-section of the vein so that cross-sectional area and flow are preserved. On colour-duplex the compression picture is often less evident than at phlebography and it is very seldom associated with an increased venous flow velocity which is indicative of stenosis. It is therefore possible that phlebography overestimates the problem. In our series of 175 patients (131 females; mean age 37.3 ± 12 years), referred because of 'inexplicable' distal left foot and/or leg oedema but with an otherwise apparently normal venous system, colour-duplex indicated some degree of compression (increased flow velocity) at the proximal iliac vein in 57 (32.6%) patients. In 22 (12.6%) of these, the cross-section of the vein was reduced by at least 50% with accompanying increased flow velocity. In seven young females (4%) there was almost complete occlusion. Therefore, a total of 36.6% of patients who present with unilateral swelling may have some degree of compression associated with postural or permanent obstruction.

Non-invasive studies (ultrasound, particularly colour-duplex) are the investigations of choice though CT or MR scans may also reveal and correctly localize the level of obstruction. Phlebography is useful but it tends, as already indicated, to overestimate compression.

In some subjects the compression is more marked and may be associated with a band or adhesion at the proximal end of the left common iliac vein. Compression at this level has also been considered to be a possible cause of venous thrombosis which is more frequent in the left leg.

The presence of recurrent oedema in the distal leg or foot may in some subjects require surgical treatment or stenting of the affected segment. In some instances of severe obstruction the vein may be dissected to eliminate constricting bands or adhesions, divided and re-anastomosed end-to-end in front of the artery or reimplanted into the inferior vena cava.

LYMPHATIC CAUSES OF A SWOLLEN LIMB

GENERAL CONSIDERATIONS

Lymphoedema is caused by abnormal pooling and stagnation of interstitial fluid because of either (primarily) a developmental abnormality of lymphatics or (secondarily) obstruction consequent on a disease process. Whatever the cause, the pathophysiological mechanism is the same in all instances. *Primary lymphoedema* (**Figure 12.2**) may appear clinically early in life or not until some years have elapsed.

Secondary lymphoedema (**Figure 12.3**) may be the result of filariasis, other infections, neoplasia, radiation injury, insect bites, surgical excision of lymph nodes or simple limb inactivity from paralysis.

DIAGNOSIS

Primary lymphoedema may, as already mentioned, be present at birth (congenital lymphoedema) but more often becomes obvious in the second or third decades (*lymphoedema praecox or early lymphoedema*). *Milroy's disease* is a chronic hereditary lymphoedema with very early onset (at, or near birth). In a small percentage of cases, it develops after the age of 35–40 into *lymphoedema tarda*. Lymphatic hypoplasia is present in some 50% of patients, varicose dilatation in 20–30% and aplasia in less than 15%. It has been suggested that any kind of lymphatic obstruction may be acquired but, independent of the underlying anatomical problem, the functional result of lymphatic obstruction is pooling in the interstitial space and increased interstitial pressure. The lymphatics dilate, making

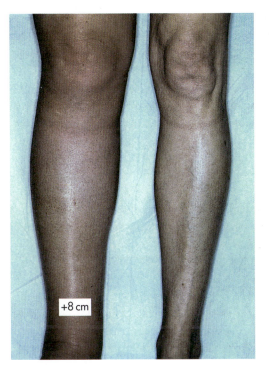

Figure 12.2 Primary lymphoedema in a young woman.

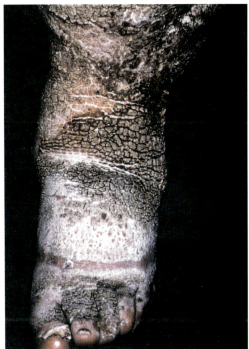

Figure 12.3 Elephantiasis of a limb in secondary, chronic lymphoedema.

their valves incompetent. Because valves are essential to promote proximal flow, incompetence of these aggravates the accumulation of interstitial fluid. The chronic presence of unremoved interstitial proteins leads to inflammation and fibrosis, interstitial compression and further obstruction. High levels of interstitial proteins increase the risk of bacterial infection. In primary lymphoedema, the swelling is initially limited to the tissues superficial to the deep fascia.

Lymphoedema praecox predominantly affects young women and begins at puberty. The first sign is a puffiness or swelling over the dorsum of the foot or at the ankle, made worse by long periods of standing or sitting. The swelling is often initially unilateral but in some subjects may be bilateral from the outset. Eventually half of all patients develop bilateral disease. The oedema slowly advances proximally so that after 1–2 years the entire limb may be involved. The swelling becomes progressively more severe and though it may initially show some pitting eventually fails to do so. Leg elevation and bed rest are eventually ineffective for its control. The subcutaneous tissues become thickened and the limb permanently enlarged. The chief complaints are of the serious disfiguration and a heavy uncomfortable limb. There is also some loss of sensation without pain, unless lymphangitis occurs.

The onset of secondary lymphoedema depends on the cause but the course of the process is similar to that of the primary form. Repeated episodes of infection cause progressive further closure of the lymphatics, so worsening the condition.

Lymphangiography and lymphoscintigraphy usually demonstrate the level and the extent of primary or secondary lymphatic obstruction (see p. 47).

DIFFERENTIAL DIAGNOSIS

Lymphoedema is easily differentiated from the peripheral swelling which occurs in systemic conditions such as heart failure and liver or renal disease, in that the oedema of the latter is bilateral, soft and pitting. Chronic venous insufficiency rarely causes a diagnostic problem because very often varicosities are present. Furthermore, the swelling of lymphoedema is generally painless, rubbery and non-pitting and decreases little if at all with leg elevation or a night's rest. By contrast, that of chronic venous insufficiency is soft and initially pits though in the later stages it becomes more firm. Associated skin pigmentation, dermatitis and eventually ulceration also suggest venous insufficiency. Recurrent lymphangitis and cellulitis are more frequent in lymphoedema. Some degree of lymphatic impairment or true lymphoedema may exist in patients with a postphlebitic limb. Where there is doubt on clinical examination, differential diagnosis is based on non-invasive investigation and occasionally on venography and lymphoscintigraphy though lymphangiography is only rarely necessary.

Obesity lymphoedema

Some degree of lymphatic impairment and oedema is also often observed in very obese subjects. However, the condition is partially or totally reversible if a significant loss of weight and increased exercise can be achieved. By contrast, most patients with true lymphoedema are very rarely obese.

Factitious oedema

A rare cause of diagnostic difficulty is self-induced oedema, usually of the upper extremity, by the clandestine application of a tight band. The underlying psychological abnormality is unclear and probably varies from patient to patient. The condition can be quite hard to detect but careful observation will usually ultimately reveal the device used and occasionally a circumferential mark on the skin at the site of constriction.

COMPLICATIONS

Infection

The uncontrolled progression of lymphoedema leads to thickening and hyperkeratosis of the skin. Cellulitis and lymphangitis may recur, even after minor trauma and are the most frequent complications. Swelling, erythema, pain and occasionally systemic signs of infection may be present. With a sluggish lymph flow the infection tends to diffuse more rapidly along the lymphatics the clinical indication of which is the diagnostic red streaks in the skin. The haemolytic streptococcus is frequently present in such infections.

Lymphangiosarcoma, an uncommon neoplasm which originates from lymphatic endothelium, may be a late complication—most commonly with postmastectomy lymphoedema of the arm. The clinical features are multiple macular or papular lesions in the skin or subcutaneous tissue though a large ulcerating mass may be present. Spread is rapid and the prognosis very poor.

CONTROL AND TREATMENT

Continued, aggressive and careful control of the oedema is the key to limit the number of complications and the progression of the condition. The prevention of recurrent infection is also very important. When oedema control and treatment are planned and used in the very early stages before fibrosis occurs, the results are satisfactory.

Physical treatment and non-operative management

In most patients with early disease, swelling is effectively controlled with physical measures. Periodic elevation during the day and sleeping with the leg 20–30 cm above the heart should be routine. Elastic compression stockings are used as much as possible during the day and should include the entire leg. Pneumatic, sequential compression (**Figure 12.4a**) is very useful but many patients find it difficult to use for the 2–3 hours daily needed to obtain good results. However, limited success at a very low cost may be obtained with the sequential compression device (SCD) generally used for prophylaxis of deep vein thrombosis (**Figure 12.4b**). The equivalent lymphatic sequential compression device is more effective but much more expensive. Simple one-chamber devices (Flowtron) are also effective. The best results are obtained with sequential compression applied in the evening before or during sleep. Restriction of dietary sodium may be considered in some patients but to use diuretics in true lymphoedema is of very questionable value.

Skin care is important to prevent infections. If repeated episodes occur, patients must be treated with specific antibiotics, recalling

Figure 12.4 (a) The Lympha-Press device for pneumatic segmental compression used in the treatment of lymphoedema. A sequential compression device (b) can be used as an alternative.

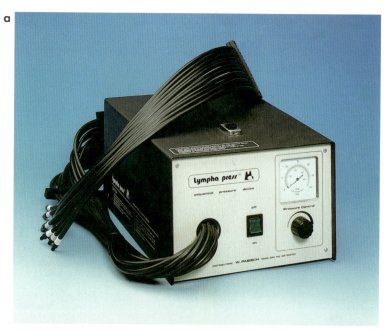

a

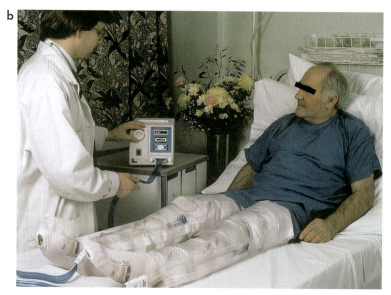

b

the fact that the most common organism is usually a streptococcus. Strenuous, continuous physical exercise in suitable young subjects is very beneficial.

The use of devices (ovens) which increase local temperature promotes interstitial protein degradation and, because the molecules which result are smaller, these are removed faster from the interstitial space. The rate of progression of the oedema decreases and the skin becomes softer. However, this type of treatment has not been widely evaluated and there are no safety data to indicate whether or not it may further damage the lymphatic system.

Repeated manual lymphatic drainage when performed by expert and specialized staff may be very effective in the early phases and also offers a good palliative solution for more advanced patients.

Surgical treatment

Surgical treatment is indicated only in a very limited number (10–15%) of patients. Indications for surgery are:

◆ very impaired limb function or appearance of deformity, excess size and weight;
◆ severe pain;
◆ repeated episodes of infections (cellulitis, lymphangitis);
◆ neoplastic development (lymphangiosarcoma).

Many patients are young women for whom cosmetic considerations are important but this is hardly ever the only indication for surgery and usually some degree of functional impairment must also be present.

Excisional procedures remove the thickened subcutaneous tissues and resurface the limb by covering the deep fascia with split skin derived either from the area removed or elsewhere in the body. Several procedures have been described. A reduction in size may be achieved but none of the techniques is really satisfactory because extensive scarring, sensory loss and some degree of persistent swelling is usually observed.

Direct procedures endeavour to increase lymph flow and drainage by relieving lymphatic obstruction. Some transfer normal lymphatic channels from a healthy area into a lymphoedematous one. In Thompson's operation, longitudinal flaps of dermis are folded beneath the muscles along the medial and lateral side of the limbs to produce new lymphatic connections between the altered superficial dermal lymphatics and the normal deep system. Clinical results may be good but the presence of new lymphatics has never been shown. Omental flaps may also be used but have been less successful. In the enteromesenteric bridge method which applies bowel to a transected lymph node, new lymphatic connections have been shown between inguinal lymph nodes and the gut and the long-term results may be remarkably satisfactory. However, these methods require extensive dissectio.. and should be used only in patients with pressing indications for surgical correction.

Microvascular surgery has made new surgical techniques available. Lymphovenous anastomosis (**Figure 12.5**) and other methods have been used but prospective studies which have analysed results obtained with these methods are not available.

Figure 12.5 Two types of lymphovenous anastomosis.

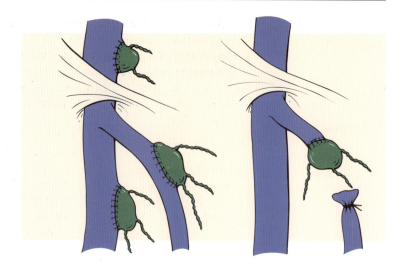

PROGNOSIS   Untreated, lymphoedema progresses to produce increasingly severe disability and disfiguration. The enlarged, heavy extremity becomes unusable and recurrent infection adds to the patient's problems. Most benefit from a carefully planned oedema control programme consonant with their lifestyle and social needs. The limited experience with surgery does not clearly indicate its benefits and prospective studies are needed.

BIBLIOGRAPHY

Borel Rinkes IH, deJongste AB. Lymphangiosarcoma in chronic lymphedema: reports of 3 cases and review of the literature. *Acta Chir Scand* 1986; **152**: 227.

Browse NL. The diagnosis and management of primary lymphedema. *J Vasc Surg* 1986; **3**: 181.

Browse NL, Stewart G. Lymphedema: pathophysiology and classification. *J Cardiovasc Surg* 1985; **26**: 91.

Christenson JT, Hamad MM, Shawa NJ. Primary lymphedema of the leg: relationship between subcutaneous tissue pressure, intramuscular pressure, and venous function. *Lymphology* 1985; **18**: 86.

Collins SP *et al*. Abnormalities of lymphatic drainage in lower extremities: a lymphoscintigraphic study. *J Vasc Surg* 1989; **9**: 145.

Cooney TG, Reuler JB. The swollen leg. *West J Med* 1985; **142**: 405.

Dodd H, Cockett FB. *The Pathology and Surgery of the Veins of the Lower Limbs*. London: Churchill Livingstone, 1976.

Gloviczki P *et al*. Non-invasive evaluation of the swollen extremity: experience with 190 lymphoscintigraphic examinations. *J Vasc Surg* 1989; **9**: 83.

Golueke PJ *et al*. Lymphoscintigraphy to confirm the clinical diagnosis of lymphedema. *J Vasc Surg* 1989; **1**: 306.

Hadjis NS *et al*. The role of CT in the diagnosis of primary lymphedema of the lower limb. *Am J Roentgenol* 1985; **144**: 361.

Huang GK *et al*. Microlymphaticovenous anastomosis in the treatment of lower limb obstructive lymphedema: analysis of 91 cases. *Plast Reconstr Surg* 1985; **76**: 671.

Hurst PAE *et al*. The long-term results of the enteromesenteric bridge operation in the treatment of primary lymphoedema. *Br J Surg* 1985; **72**: 272.

Lewis JM, Wald ER. Lymphedema praecox. *J Pediatr* 1984; **104**: 641.

Norberg B. The swollen leg. (Editorial) *Acta Med Scand* 1988; **224**: 1.

Qvarfordt P *et al*. Intramuscular pressure, venous function, and muscle blood flow in patients with lymphedema of the leg. *Lymphology* 1983; **16**: 139.

Richmond DM, O'Donnell TF Jr, Zelikovski A. Sequential pneumatic compression for lymphedema: a controlled trial. *Arch Surg* 1985; **120**: 1116.

Savage RC. The surgical management of lymphedema. *Surg Gynecol Obstet* 1985; **160**: 283.

Smeltzer DM, Stickler GB, Schirger A. Primary lymphedema in children and adolescents: a follow-up study and review. *Pediatrics* 1985; **76**: 206.

Stewart G *et al*. Isotope lymphography: a new method of investigating the role of the lymphatics in chronic limb oedema. *Br J Surg* 1985; **72**: 906.

Wolfe JH. The prognosis and possible cause of severe primary lymphoedema. *Ann R Coll Surg Engl* 1984; **66**: 251.

Zelikovski A, Haddad M, Reiss R. The 'Lympha-Press' intermittent sequential pneumatic device for treatment of lymphedema; five years of clinical experience. *J Cardiovasc Surg* 1986; **27**: 288.

Genital disorders involving the venous system

VARICOCELE

GENERAL CONSIDERATIONS

Varicocele is thought to be the result of incompetence of the valves in the spermatic and testicular veins so that there is an increased venous pressure in the pampiniform plexus with consequential dilatation and tortuosity. Ninety per cent of varicoceles are on the left side where the termination of the spermatic vein into the left renal vein allows more direct transmission of retrograde pressure along the incompetent vein to the contents of the scrotum. Dilated veins may be present without valvular incompetence in which circumstance by definition there is not a varicocele. Incompetence may also exist without dilatation.

DIAGNOSIS

Clinically overt varicocele is easy to diagnose and evaluate. The patient may complain of a dragging scrotal sensation; the left hemiscrotum and testis are enlarged; and, when the patient stands, dilated veins are visible and palpable. A mild varicocele may be asymptomatic and difficult to detect. Varicocele, clinical or subclinical, is considered to be an important cause of male infertility.

The diagnosis of varicocele is now confirmed by ultrasound. B-mode scanning indicates the presence of dilated veins, increasing in size during a Valsalva manoeuvre or on standing. Duplex or colour-duplex scanning visualize the veins and can demonstrate transient reflux as intra-abdominal pressure is increased: it is best shown and can be as far as the spermatic plexus with the patient supine, fully relaxed and performing (**Figure 13.1**). **Figure 13.2** shows the dilated veins with, in the tracing, reflux initiated by a Valsalva manoeuvre. When reflux cannot be demonstrated in the supine position, the test may be repeated with the patient standing.

Retrograde phlebography is also still widely used to demonstrate varicocele.

Figure 13.1 Colour-duplex ultrasound of a patient with varicocele during a Valsalva manoeuvre. Reflux into the spermatic plexus is shown in red and extends into the veins surrounding the testis (right image).

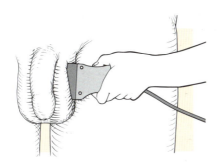

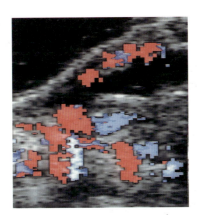

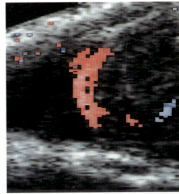

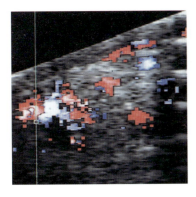

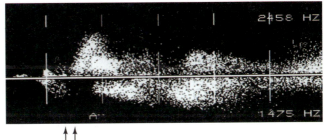

Figure 13.2 Combined colour-duplex and tracing (arrows) during a Valsalva manoeuvre.

MANAGEMENT *Symptomatic varicocele*, including that associated with infertility, is usually treated surgically by ligation of the spermatic vein at or above the internal inguinal ring. The procedure can be done laparoscopically.

Recurrent varicocele and *asymptomatic varicocele associated with significant reflux (>3 seconds) on colour-duplex* may be treated with transfemoral catheterization of the left spermatic vein and retrograde injection of sclerosing agents. Alternatively, occlusion of the spermatic vein may be produced with a detachable balloon inserted via the femoral vein.

The long-term results are usually very satisfactory.

THE PELVIC CONGESTION SYNDROME (PCS)

GENERAL CONSIDERATIONS This syndrome is sometimes unrecognized or not clearly defined because many patients are treated by different specialists for the two main problems involved—pelvic pain and vulvar varicosities. Vulvar varicose veins are a relatively common disorder sometimes associated with pelvic pain. The genesis of vulvar varicose veins has been regarded as equivalent to that of the post-thrombotic syndrome in the legs. They are common during pregnancy but usually disappear after delivery. However, during or following a pregnancy some of the tributaries of the internal iliac veins occlude and outflow obstruction results. In particular, the sudden appearance of vulvar varicose veins during the third or fourth month of a second or third pregnancy may indicate thrombosis in the pelvic veins. Persistence and increase in size and extent—including spread to the posterior part of the leg and thigh—may then take place in any pregnancy that follows.

PCS is characterized by pain of variable intensity which is worse premenstrually and greatly increased by fatigue, standing and especially during intercourse. These symptoms are often associated with the presence of vulvar varicosities. Also 'broad ligament varicocele' has been associated with chronic pelvic pain in multiparous women. Pelvic varicosities also occur when the ovarian veins are congenitally incompetent, causing a situation which is analogous to scrotal varicocele in men.

DIAGNOSIS On examination of patients with PCS, atypical veins are present on the back of the thigh arising from the posterior vulvar area. The vulvar varicosities may be in communication with the long saphenous vein which fills from the posterior vulvar veins.

Ovarian varicocele may be diagnosed by ultrasound, or phlebography. A congested ovary may be shown by ultrasound and the presence of reflux in the ovarian veins may be observed by the use of colour-duplex during a Valsalva manoeuvre but this finding is inconstant. The dilated ovarian vein may be demonstrated by direct vulvar venography or by retrograde phlebography. It is important to exclude other inflammatory conditions such as inflammatory bowel disease, pelvic inflammatory disease and endometriosis. Vertebral problems causing neural compression and pain should also be considered.

MANAGEMENT

The usual first line of treatment is conservative by suppression of ovarian function. Retroperitoneal ligation of the veins, ovariectomy or even hysterectomy may, however, be required. Sclerotherapy of the vulvar veins with 3% STD has also been used by Hobbs with good results. Retrograde catheterization and sclerosis of the ovarian vein has also been attempted.

If it is untreated, PCS tends to disappear after the menopause.

HAEMORRHOIDS

GENERAL CONSIDERATIONS

The closure of the anal canal by 'cushions' of tissue that contain venous plexuses is a normal state and it is only when the cushions become enlarged and produce symptoms and signs that haemorrhoids are said to be present and may require treatment (**Figure 13.3**).

Figure 13.3 The usual arrangement of primary and secondary internal haemorrhoids. The anal canal is seen with the patient in the lithotomy position.

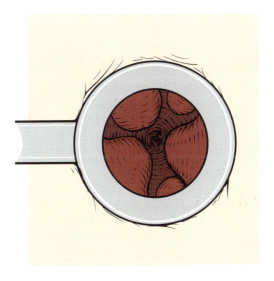

The old classification into *internal* and *external* haemorrhoids is now obsolete. Increase in the size of cushions which are part of the inferior haemorrhoidal venous plexus is associated with bulging which affects the terminal mucosa and adjacent skin of the anal canal. The mass so formed has both mucosa and skin overlying it and whether or not the resulting 'haemorrhoids' prolapse through the anus so as to be seen externally is a complex function of the degree of straining that takes place and the tone of the anal sphincter. Haemorrhoids may be said to be internal when they do not prolapse and intero-external when they do. For the anatomical reasons discussed in Chapter 1, the anal cushions are at the junction of the systemic and splanchnic venous systems and drainage may be into either system depending on the venous dynamics of the two.

Hypertrophied anal cushions become symptomatic for a variety of reasons, including straining in the squatting position which increases venous pressure, so distending the veins and predisposing to protrusion and bleeding. Other factors considered to be important are chronic constipation, pregnancy, obesity and a low-fibre diet which leads to greater straining and therefore increased venous pressure during defaecation. The latter is particularly the case if the individual is obsessively concerned about complete emptying of the bowel.

In spite of all these observations, the underlying cause of hypertrophy of the anal cushions and the development of haemorrhoids remains uncertain. There is no evidence to support the concept that it might be analogous to lower limb varicose veins, though this is an attractive hypothesis given that there are valves in the haemorrhoidal venous system.

DIAGNOSIS

Patients may say they have 'haemorrhoids' merely because they have anal symptoms. Severe pain is present in two circumstances:

♦ a localized thrombosis in the perianal skin, the so-called 'thrombosed external pile' which has nothing to do with changes in the anal cushions;
♦ thrombosis of large haemorrhoids that have prolapsed through the anal sphincter at defaecation and become trapped externally when the sphincter closes.

Bleeding is usually the first indication of problems. The blood is bright red, not mixed with the stools, and is variable in quantity. Recurrent bleeding may lead to anaemia. Enlargement of the cushions without prolapse is the initial stage (first degree haemorrhoids). As a further increase in size takes place, prolapse on defaecation occurs, followed by spontaneous reduction (second degree) while later the patient may be forced to replace them manually (third degree). Finally, prolapse may be permanent (fourth degree).

On examination in the early stage, little may be found other than an increased size of the cushions at the anal verge. As the condition develops, the anal verge may protrude and mucosa becomes visible, first on straining and later in the resting state because the mass is now intero-external. On digital rectal examination, uncomplicated haemorrhoids cannot be palpated and are not associated with tenderness. Anoscopic examination may reveal evidence of bleeding and a subjective impression that the cushions are enlarged is obtained. Gentle straining by the patient may be associated with prolapse. Proctosigmoidoscopy is needed to exclude inflammatory or neoplastic disease at a higher level.

DIFFERENTIAL DIAGNOSIS

The most common feature of haemorrhoids—rectal bleeding— occurs also in colorectal malignancy, adenomatous polyps, diverticular disease, and inflammatory disorders. If there is any doubt after clinical assessment and proctosigmoidoscopy, more detailed investigation is needed, particularly in older patients, by barium enema, colonoscopy and mucosal biopsy. Rectal prolapse is differentiated from prolapsing haemorrhoids by the appearance of a complete circle of protruding bowel with concentric mucosal folds; the full thickness of the wall is involved and can be detected by digital palpation.

Haemorrhoids and rectal prolapse may coexist. Other perianal lesions and anorectal tumours are characteristic in their appearance. The *thrombosed external haemorrhoid* is described in the following section. The presence of external skin tags may indicate previous thrombosis of external haemorrhoids while the presence of a midline sentinel tag may be the external evidence of the presence of an anal fissure.

COMPLICATIONS

Occasionally prolapsing haemorrhoids become irreducible—a consequence of congestion from a tight anal sphincter, oedema and/or thrombosis of the veins within them. There is severe pain and the mucosa and, rarely, adjacent skin may necrose. A very few patients with thrombosed haemorrhoids develop portal pyaemia and multiple liver abscesses. Anaemia is a relatively common complication. It is said that in patients with portal hypertension bleeding may be very profuse because haemorrhoids may be part of the enlarged portosystemic communications. However, the evidence for this is not very strong.

MANAGEMENT

The aim of treatment is to make the patient asymptomatic and the method used is based on the clinical presentation.

Conservative medical treatment

A diet high in fibre, increased water intake and hydrophilic agents to increase faecal bulk are used in first and second degree haemorrhoids.

Injection treatment (sclerotherapy)

Injection treatment may be added to the medical regimen in patients with troublesome bleeding or those with early prolapse. A haemorrhoidal needle is used to inject through an anoscope above the mucocutaneous junction. The sclerosing agent (e.g. 5% phenol in vegetable oil) is injected submucosally into the loose areolar tissue above the haemorrhoids. Inflammation and scarring occur after injection and reduce the bulk of the lesion.

Rubber band ligation

This is used for much enlarged and prolapsing haemorrhoids. With an anoscope the redundant mucosa above the haemorrhoidal plexus is grasped and advanced through a special ligator. The rubber band causes ischaemic necrosis, followed by fibrosis and fixation of the tissues. After treatment, pain may be very severe and require the removal of the band.

Cryosurgery

Cryosurgery destroys haemorrhoids by cold necrosis using a cryoprobe (CO_2 or N_2O). The method is not very satisfactory because delayed wound healing may occur.

Surgery (haemorrhoidectomy)

Surgery is used for patients with severe, chronic symptoms and third or fourth degree lesions. These subjects are often anaemic. The procedure consists of excision of the redundant tissue which contains the venous dilatations, with conservation of normal mucosa and skin. The underlying sphincter must be left undamaged. Surgical treatment may also be done using a laser.

Other methods

Other methods include anal dilatation (to disrupt fibrous bands in the anal canal and possibly to reduce sphincter tone), infrared photocoagulation and bipolar diathermy. Their rate of success is not clear.

THROMBOSED EXTERNAL HAEMORRHOID

The condition is characterized by a painful, tense, bluish mass beneath the skin at the mucocutaneous junction, and is caused by thrombosis in the subcutaneous external haemorrhoidal vein of the anal canal. Some consider it to be the outcome of bleeding into the dense mesh of connective tissue in the region—a perianal haematoma—but the lesion has been shown to have an endothelial lining and therefore almost certainly is a true thrombosis. The condition usually follows a sudden increase in abdominal pressure (heavy lifting, coughing, sneezing, straining during defaecation), but may occur spontaneously. It generally affects young healthy subjects, is not directly related to disorders of the anal cushions and must be distinguished from prolapsed haemorrhoids because treatment is completely different.

Immediate relief may be obtained if the patient is seen within the first 48 hours, by evacuation of the thrombus or complete excision. An ellipse of skin should also be removed to prevent re-formation of the underlying clot. When the thrombus has become organized, conservative measures are more appropriate.

BIBLIOGRAPHY

Hargreave TB. Varicocele—a clinical enigma. *Br J Urol* 1993; **72**: 401.

Hobbs JT. The pelvic congestion syndrome. *The Practitioner* 1976; **216**: 529.

Hobbs JT. The pelvic congestion syndrome. *Br J Hosp Update* 1990; **43**: 200.

Keighley MRB, Williams NS. *Surgery of the Anus, Rectum and Colon.* London: WB Saunders, 1993.

CHAPTER 14

Less common disorders involving veins

KLIPPEL–TRENAUNAY (LATERAL VENOUS) SYNDROME

GENERAL CONSIDERATIONS In early intrauterine life the lower limb has a ventral vascular system (the primitive femoral artery and veins) and a dorsal or sciatic system. During the second month the femoral system continues to develop while the sciatic system atrophies almost completely. However, in some subjects the sciatic system persists, generating a large group of venous anomalies included under the name of *Klippel–Trenaunay syndrome (KTS)* or *lateral venous anomalies*. A similar phenomenon can occur in the arm but is six times less common. In one in ten patients the syndrome may be bilateral or occur in both the upper and lower limb of the same side. In the lower limb angiomas, varicose veins and hypertrophy in soft tissues and bone affect the lateral and posterior surface of the limb and often extend proximally into the buttock and the vascular territory of the internal iliac artery and vein. There are three clinical variants of the KTS as follows.

Type 1 is the fully developed anomaly with skin angiomas over the entire, lateral side of the leg from the foot up to the buttock. Deep to the skin and spreading through subcutaneous tissue, muscle and occasionally bone there is diffuse angiomatosis. Sometimes the venous spaces flow into the internal iliac vein through a series of large abnormal venous channels. Precapillary arteriovenous fistulas may also be present with low-resistance arterial flow associated with increased growth of all components of the limb so that the leg is both longer and its girth increased. Involvement of the pelvic structures may be associated with recurrent rectal haemorrhages and very large haemorrhoids have also been described.

Type 2 is a venous anomaly only, without arteriovenous communication or increase in limb size. Diffuse cavernous haemangioma is the most important feature and consists of large and small venous spaces which lack the well defined wall of normal large veins. There is often a direct communication with the internal iliac vein and large deep to superficial communicating vessels are found. A diffuse, patchy, capillary haemangioma is present over the lateral and posterior surface of the leg and thigh. Phleboliths and localized thrombi may be found. Heaviness and disfiguration are the most common complaints. Chronic venous insufficiency may develop if the major incompetent veins are left untreated and recurrent DVT and PE are possible.

Type 3 is the minor form of the syndrome presenting as diffuse varicose veins on the lateral side of the thigh and leg. Often no haemangiomas or only little patches are present. Most cases have diffuse, small, tortuous varicosities usually without evidence of long or short saphenous incompetence.

DIAGNOSIS In most cases this is purely clinical. It is possible to evaluate the extent of the vascular anomalies in the deep tissues with MRI. Non-invasive investigations (duplex and colour-duplex) may confirm the presence of an arteriovenous communication. Phlebography is used to study the deep veins which may be absent or underdeveloped as their role is taken over by the abnormal ones. If there is evidence of widespread arteriovenous shunting, angiography gives useful anatomical information and it is sometimes possible to embolize the most important arterial anomalies at the same procedure.

In children it is advisable to investigate for the presence of other possible developmental anomalies and to advise the orthopaedic unit of a possible different development of the affected limb so that the patient may be treated at the appropriate time.

MANAGEMENT

In *Type 1 KTS* management is generally conservative. Patients must be advised to avoid trauma and use compression and elevation from an early stage. Surgery is usually indicated to ligate the larger venous sites, communicating veins or large varices which contribute to the chronic increase in venous pressure. Large incisions in or over haemangiomatous areas may result in chronic ulceration which proves very difficult to heal. When the increase in growth rate of the limb is excessive, embolization of some of the feeding vessels may be considered. There is no definitive standard treatment for this condition because of the variability of the clinical picture. Therefore surgical treatment should be considered on an individual basis.

Types 2 and 3 KTS are managed with compression and selective surgery, often repeated, of the most important venous anomalies. The same precautions about siting incisions in normal skin have to be taken if delayed healing is to be avoided. Sclerotherapy, when possible, may help to control diffuse varicosity. Amputation of a most severely affected limb has been reported but is now rarely needed.

PROGNOSIS

The variability of signs and symptoms between patients is large. Most patients have a normal, active life. The approach should be optimistic because conservative treatment and selective surgery are effective in most patients to control the course of KTS.

HAEMANGIOMAS

GENERAL CONSIDERATIONS

The most readily accepted aetiological concept is that haemangiomas are a failure to complete angiogenesis during which primitive collections of undifferentiated blood sinuses mature into the arteries, capillaries and veins. In consequence the lesions contain varying amounts of each component of the vascular system with large venous-like lakes often predominant. An element of arteriovenous communication may coexist. Haemangiomas which present at birth may, on occasion, continue to differentiate and disappear as a consequence of this process and associated thrombosis.

Types of haemangioma and their management

Capillary haemangioma may be superficial or the visible part of a more extensive deep haemangioma. Removal of the lesion is often considered for cosmetic reasons or when it causes repeated bleeding or is associated with infection. If possible such surgical treatment should be complete excision of the lesion including any overlying intact skin because incisions and wounds in the skin over a haemangioma heal poorly.

In infants who are not threatened by complications, an initial conservative approach is used to see if the lesion may undergo spontaneous regression.

Cavernous haemangiomas are usually deep masses containing venous spaces which may involve all tissues including bone. MRI reveals the extent of such lesions. Those that are diffuse are usually treated conservatively as surgical excision is often impossible. Ligation or sclerotherapy of some venous channels may, however, be beneficial and be considered on an individual basis.

An apparently *localized lesion* may appear to have only a few large venous sinuses which could be successfully removed surgically. However, most appear more localized than they are and the surgical approach may be more challenging than anticipated. Therefore careful visualization of the lesion before surgery is essential.

ABNORMAL ARTERIOVENOUS COMMUNICATIONS (FISTULAS)

GENERAL CONSIDERATIONS

Abnormal arteriovenous communications (fistulas) may be congenital or acquired. Abnormal arteriovenous communications occur in many diseases and may affect vessels of all sizes. Their effects depend upon their size. In *congenital fistulas,* the systemic effect is often not great, because, though the communications are often numerous and diffuse, they are small and the amount of blood passing through them not large. Larger *acquired fistulas* tend to increase in size, often rapidly. A low-resistance fistula results in an increase in cardiac output which if allowed to persist may cause cardiac dilatation and failure. Arteriovenous fistulas have also been conjectured to be one of the abnormalities underlying varicose veins but this hypothesis does not receive much contemporary support. Small congenital fistulas are often observed in infancy or childhood and as with haemangiomas may undergo spontaneous regression. When a limb is involved, muscle mass or bone length may be increased. Arteriovenous malformations frequently involve the brain, visceral organs or lungs. Gastrointestinal haemorrhage may occur. Pulmonary lesions cause polycythaemia, clubbing and cyanosis.

Acquired fistulas usually result from injuries that produce artificial connections between adjacent arteries and veins and may be the result of trauma or disease. Penetrating injuries are the most common cause but fistulas are also occasionally seen after blunt trauma.

Iatrogenic arteriovenous fistulas after arteriography are becoming increasingly common. *Connective tissue disorders* (e.g. Ehlers–Danlos syndrome), erosion of *an atherosclerotic* or *mycotic arterial aneurysm* into adjacent veins, communication with an *arterial prosthetic graft* and neoplastic invasion are other causes. Finally, a rare but dramatic cause of arteriovenous fistula is combined injury to the aorta and inferior vena cava or to the iliac arteries and veins during *surgical excision of a herniated nucleus pulposus* by the dorsal approach.

CLINICAL FINDINGS

Symptoms and signs

The time of onset and the presence or absence of associated disease should be determined. A typical continuous machinery murmur can be heard over most fistulas and is often associated with a palpable thrill and locally increased skin temperature. Proximally, the arteries and veins dilate and the pulse distal to the lesion diminishes. The limb, distal to the communication, may be cooler. There may be varicose veins or signs of venous insufficiency. Tachycardia occurs in some subjects as a consequence of increased cardiac output and left ventricular overload.

When the fistula is occluded by manual compression or by compression with an ultrasound probe, the pulse rate tends to slow (Branham's sign).

Imaging

Non-invasive investigations (duplex and colour-duplex scanning) are very effective in imaging fistulas and their connections; occasionally it is also possible to quantify blood flow. A typical low-resistance waveform (with high diastolic component) and high systolic velocity are demonstrated in most patients (**Figure 14.1**). In the most severe cases the venous flow is completely modified from a waveform phasic with respiration to a continuous high velocity pattern.

Figure 14.1
Arteriovenous fistula
(AVF). PTV = popliteal
vein.

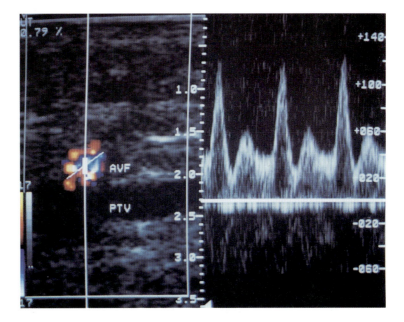

Magnetic resonance imaging (MRI) has an important role in the evaluation and follow-up of arteriovenous malformations. The precise delineation of larger arteriovenous fistulas is undertaken with selective arteriography and the procedure is indicated when surgery or embolization are planned.

MANAGEMENT

Only some arteriovenous connections require treatment. Small peripheral fistulas may be a cosmetic problem but, if there is not a severe associated haemodynamic disorder, a conservative approach is indicated. Also, many fistulas are too diffuse, too small or too deep to be surgically accessible.

The indications for surgery or radiological intervention include external bleeding, expanding false aneurysm, severe venous or arterial insufficiency, important cosmetic deformity and, in a limited number of patients only, heart failure. Many fistulas are now managed by the interventional radiologist with arterial embolization under angiographic control. Several types of embolic material have been used such as Gelfoam™, blood clots, glass beads and autologous muscle tissue.

Good results have been documented with arteriovenous malformations in different anatomical areas. Intracranial arteriovenous malformations and all fistulas of the head and neck appear better suited for this form of therapy which has the advantage of being repeatable.

Surgical treatment theoretically includes ligation of all major feeding arteries and draining veins. However, the procedure is most often incomplete and recurrence after some time is likely, particularly in congenital malformations. Amputation of the extremity, *en bloc* resection of the tissue including the fistula and repair of the fistula by reconstruction of the involved arteries and veins are other possibilities. Oversewing the defects in the artery and vein is curative for post-arteriography fistulas.

Congenital arteriovenous fistulas are amenable to surgical management only when *en bloc* resection of all tissue involved in the fistula can be accomplished. When the fistulous connections involve substantial portions of an extremity, local arterial ligation is invariably followed by recurrence and thus only temporary palliation can be expected. Amputation may be a last resort to control unmanageable peripheral fistulas.

PROGNOSIS

The results of therapy vary according to the extent, location and type of fistula. In general, traumatic fistulas have a favourable prognosis and technically they are often corrected without problems. The reverse is true for congenital fistulas. The multiplicity of connections make them difficult to control and recurrence inevitable.

PRIMARY AORTOCAVAL FISTULA

This is a special example of an arteriovenous connection found between an abdominal aortic aneurysm and the inferior vena cava in 1–2% of patients treated for abdominal aortic aneurysm and in 5–6% of those with a rupture. The fistula is often undiagnosed before operation for ruptured aneurysm but specific signs such as a pulsating abdominal mass and high output heart failure may be present. Pulmonary embolism is rare. However, aortocaval fistulas do not necessarily draw attention to themselves, especially if the clinical situation is complex and they usually come as a surprise to the surgeon.

Surgery is the only possible course of action for most patients with aortocaval fistulas. Surgical repair after careful dissection of the iliac veins and the cava is very rarely possible. Digital control of the arteriovenous communication and endoaneurysmal repair of the fistula has been accomplished but carries a high mortality rate (35–40%) mainly because of multiple organ failure.

RENAL VEIN THROMBOSIS (RVT)

GENERAL CONSIDERATIONS

The condition occurs principally in infants and more than two-thirds present at less than a month of age. Most instances are diagnosed only at postmortem examination. The condition is thought to be related to the haemodynamics of the renal vein in very early life: low blood flow, relative polycythaemia, and high vascular resistance. Further factors are reduced fibrinolysis, increased osmolality associated with water lack, hypovolaemia, haemoconcentration and hyperviscosity, all of which may predispose to the formation of small thrombi in venous radicals which may spread to the arcuate, interlobular and renal veins. The opposite direction of spread is uncommon. Renal vein thrombosis does, however, cause renal congestion and often infarction.

SYMPTOMS AND SIGNS

Haematuria, vomiting, pallor, tachypnoea, abdominal distension, shock, oliguria and finally anuria may all be present. A sudden enlargement of one or both kidneys can be detected on clinical examination in nearly two-thirds of patients.

LABORATORY FINDINGS

Common findings are: proteinuria; microangiopathic haemolytic anaemia with red cell fragmentation; thrombocytopenia; low levels of fibrinogen, factor V and plasminogen; and increased concentration of fibrin degradation products. These signs may reflect disseminated intravascular coagulation. Urograms should not be done. The most useful tests are ultrasound imaging of the kidneys and colour-Doppler evaluation of flow in the renal veins and arteries. Isotope renography may also be useful. Venography is risky and usually unnecessary.

DIFFERENTIAL DIAGNOSIS

This must be made between RVT and haemolytic–uraemic syndrome. Perirenal haematoma, abscess, hydronephrosis, cysts and tumours may all be confused with RVT.

MANAGEMENT

Management is usually conservative and supportive, planned to correct the causative factors. Dialysis may be necessary. Anticoagulant treatment has been used but its efficacy is not clearly documented. It may be considered when there is laboratory evidence of intravascular coagulation. Surgery is rarely performed.

The mortality rate is high but is related to the underlying conditions more than to the RVT. Renal function may recover completely but scarring or atrophy of the affected kidneys may occur leading ultimately to chronic renal failure and hypertension.

Renal vein thrombosis in adults is usually a consequence of renal infection, ascending caval thrombosis or caval occlusion by a tumour thrombus. Treatment should attempt to eliminate the underlying cause. If thrombosis occurs in an infected kidney, nephrectomy is indicated. In bilateral disease, anticoagulant or thrombolytic therapy is indicated.

SPLENIC VEIN THROMBOSIS

The condition is usually the consequence of some condition in the adjacent pancreas: inflammation, trauma and extrinsic obstruction from a tumour or pseudocyst. Splenomegaly is usually present. Isolated splenic vein thrombosis with local venous hypertension leading to oesophageal varices can cause upper gastrointestinal bleeding and in such circumstances splenectomy is curative. However, many cases are not associated with bleeding varices and in these patients treatment is not indicated.

EXTENSION OF A RENAL ADENOCARCINOMA INTO THE LUMEN OF THE INFERIOR VENA CAVA

The condition is asymptomatic but may occasionally be detected on preoperative investigation. The neoplastic 'pseudo-thrombus' may be below the level of the liver (40%), retrohepatic (45%) or reach the right atrium (15%). In such circumstances the excision of the tumour should be associated with the removal of intraluminal growth. Complex procedures may be needed and cardiopulmonary bypass may have to be used.

POPLITEAL VEIN ENTRAPMENT

Entrapment of the popliteal *artery* because of anomalous anatomy (typically the insertion of one head of the gastrocnemius muscle) as a cause of ischaemic symptoms has been described. Comparable entrapment of the popliteal vein has also been postulated as a cause of venous obstruction or a predisposing factor in deep venous thrombosis. The incidence of popliteal vein compression by full knee extension in a normal population has been recently studied by duplex scanning. Knee extension produced complete obstruction in 17% of subjects and greater than 50% reduction in diameter in a further 10%. However, air plethysmography showed outflow obstruction in only a few limbs and even fewer had symptoms or signs of obstruction. Phlebographic evaluation of the popliteal vein may often show what appears to be compression which is not clinically relevant. Surgery may be very rarely indicated in a patient with symptoms and signs and with documented obstruction.

BIBLIOGRAPHY

Bryant RS, Russel EJ, Curtin JW. Combined treatment of arteriovenous malformations by transarterial microembolization and surgery. *Am Surg* 1988; **54**: 637.

Dodd H., Cockett F.B. *The Pathology and Surgery of the Veins of the Lower Limb.* Edinburgh: Churchill-Livingstone, 1975.

Gilardi G, Scorza R *et al.* Primary aortocaval fistula. *Cardiovasc Surg* 1994; **2**: 495.

Leighton Hill L. Renal vascular thrombosis. In: Oski FA *et al.*, eds. *Principles and Practice of Pediatrics.* Philadelphia: JB Lippincott Co, 1994.

Lie JT. Pathology of angiodysplasia in Klippel–Trenaunay syndrome. *Pathol Res Pract* 1988; **183**: 747.

Pearce WH *et al.* Nuclear magnetic resonance imaging: its diagnostic value in patients with congenital vascular malformations of the limbs. *J Vasc Surg* 1988; **8**: 64.

Schonbach B, Schlosser V. Pathogenesis and changes in the aetiology of arteriovenous fistulae. *Eur J Vasc Surg* 1990; **4**: 233.

Widlus DM *et al.* Congenital arteriovenous malformation: tailored embolotherapy. *Radiology* 1988; **169**: 511.

Drugs and physical treatments used in venous diseases

The drugs used for venous diseases may be divided into four main groups:

◆ drugs used for DVT prophylaxis;
◆ drugs used for DVT treatment;
◆ drugs used for venous insufficiency;
◆ drugs used for sclerotherapy.

These drugs may be classified according to their mechanisms of action (**Table 15.1**).

The most important **physical methods** used to treat venous diseases are:

◆ elastic compression stockings;
◆ bandages;
◆ pneumatic (simple or sequential) compression.

ANTICOAGULANTS   The main use of anticoagulants is to prevent thrombus formation or extension of an existing thrombus. The prevention is mainly directed to stop the progression of venous thrombi consisting of a fibrin web enmeshed with platelets and red cells. They are therefore widely used in the prevention and treatment of DVT, particularly in the leg.

Heparin   Heparin is defined as **standard** or **unfractionated** in contrast with **low-molecular-weight heparins (LMWH)**. Heparin initiates anticoagulation rapidly but has a short duration of action. For the ini-

Anticoagulants and protamine
Parenteral anticoagulants
 Heparin and low-dose subcutaneous heparin
 Low-molecular-weight heparin (LMWH)
 Ancrod
Protamine

Oral anticoagulants
 Warfarin
 Nicoumalone
 Phenindione

Antiplatelet drugs
 Aspirin
 Dipyridamole
 Ticlopidine
 Indobufen

Fibrinolytic drugs
 Anteplase (rt-PA, tissue-type plasminogen activator)
 Streptokinase
 Urokinase

Other drugs used for DVT and PE prophylaxis
 Dextran 500
 Heparinoids/antithrombotics

Venoactive drugs
 Daflon
 Centella (Centellase)
 Troxerutin
 Venoruton, Paroven

Drugs used for venous ulcerations
 Defibrotide
 Oxpentifylline

tial treatment of DVT and PE, an intravenous loading dose is followed by continuous intravenous infusion (using an infusion pump) or by intermittent subcutaneous injection. The use of intermittent intravenous injection is no longer recommended. An oral anticoagulant (usually warfarin) is started at the same time or a few hours after heparin (which needs to be continued for at least 3 days or until the oral anticoagulant has taken effect). Daily laboratory monitoring is essential. The determination of APTT (activated partial thromboplastin time) is the most widely used method.

Low-dose heparin by subcutaneous injection is widely used for preventing DVT and PE in high-risk patients (see Chapter 14).

Laboratory monitoring is not required with this standard prophylactic regimen. An **adjusted dose regimen (with monitoring)** or **LMWH** is used in major orthopaedic surgery which has an increased risk of DVT and PE.

Cautions Platelet counts must be checked in patients treated for more than 5 days. Heparin should be stopped immediately in subjects developing thrombocytopenia.

Complications Haemorrhage is the most common complication. In this case heparin treatment is usually discontinued. When a rapid action recoagulation is needed, protamine sulphate is the specific antidote to stop the action of heparin.

Contraindications Heparin is contraindicated in subjects with haemophilia, haemorrhagic disorders, thrombocytopenia, active peptic ulcer, cerebral aneurysm, severe liver disease, recent surgery of the eye or nervous system, severe hypertension and hypersensitivity to heparin.

Side effects Side effects of heparin include haemorrhage, skin necrosis, thrombocytopenia, hypersensitivity reactions, osteoporosis (after prolonged use) and alopecia.

Treatment of DVT and PE A loading intravenous injection (5000 units or 10 000 in severe PE) is administered, followed by continuous infusion (1000–2000 units/h) or by subcutaneous injection of 15 000 units every 12 hours (both adjusted daily by laboratory monitoring). In small adults and children a lower loading dose is used, 15–25 units/kg per hour intravenously or 250 units/kg every 12 hours by subcutaneous injection.

Prophylaxis of DVT and PE Prophylaxis consists of subcutaneous injection (5000 units) 2 hours before surgery then every 8–12 hours for 7 days or until the patient is ambulant. With this method, monitoring is not needed. During pregnancy (with monitoring) 10 000 units are given every 12 hours (this does not cover prevention of thrombosis of prosthetic heart valves).

   These doses are recommended by the British Society for Haematology.

Low-molecular-weight heparins (LMWHs) Low-molecular-weight heparins (LMWHs) are as effective and safe as unfractionated heparin in the prevention of DVT and PE. In orthopaedic surgery they are probably more effective. Their duration of action is longer than unfractionated heparin. They are generally used once daily and the standard prophylactic regimen does not require monitoring. The effects of LMWHs are only partially reversed by protamine. Different dosages are used with different LMWHs as the fractions in the compounds differ in quantity and quality. Also, different compounds are available in different countries. Specific instructions must be observed and prophylaxis dosage cannot be generalized. However, these compounds are used once daily for prophylaxis.

Protamine sulphate   Protamine sulphate is used to counteract the action of heparin. Side effects include flushing, hypotension and bradycardia.

Dose   Dose is by slow infusion; 1 mg neutralizes 100 units of heparin (mucous) or 80 units of heparin (lung) when given within 15 minutes of heparin administration. If a long time has elapsed since heparin administration, less protamine is required because heparin is rapidly excreted. The maximum dose is 50 mg.

Ancrod   Ancrod reduces plasma fibrinogen by cleavage of fibrin. The **indications for use** are DVT and prevention of postoperative thrombosis ('named patient' basis only).

Cautions, contraindications and side effects   These are similar to those described for heparin. Resistance may develop. Administration with dextran must be avoided.

Dose   Dose is by intravenous infusion, 2–3 units/kg over 4–12 hours (usually 6–8 hours), then, by infusion or slow intravenous injection, 2 units/kg every 12 hours. By subcutaneous injection ancrod is used for prophylaxis of DVT at the dose of 280 units immediately after surgery, then 70 units daily for 4 days (for example, for fractured femur) or 8 days (for example, for hip replacement).

The initial infusion must be slow to avoid massive intravascular formation of unstable fibrin. Response is monitored, observing clot size after the blood has been allowed to stand for 2 hours. Plasma fibrinogen concentration can also be measured directly.

Complications   The most frequent complication is haemorrhage. Because it takes 12–24 hours for haemostatic fibrinogen concentrations to be restored after stopping administration, it may be necessary to give ancrod antivenom (Arvin Antidote 0.2 ml test dose subcutaneously, followed by 0.8 ml intramuscularly and, 30 minutes later 1 ml intravenously). The antivenom may cause anaphylaxis. As an alternative, reconstituted freeze-dried fibrinogen or fresh frozen plasma may be given.

ORAL ANTICOAGULANTS (OA)

Oral anticoagulants antagonize the effects of vitamin K. They take about 48–72 hours to develop their full anticoagulant effect. When immediate anticoagulation is needed, heparin is given simultaneously. The main indications for OA are DVT and PE.

OA in pregnancy

Oral anticoagulants may damage the fetus and should not be given in the first trimester of pregnancy. Women at risk of pregnancy should stop warfarin. Oral anticoagulants also cross the placenta, causing risk of fetal haemorrhage. Therefore all anticoagulants should be avoided as far as possible during pregnancy, particularly during the first and last trimesters. Difficult decisions have to be made for women with prosthetic heart valves with a history of recent DVT or PE.

Warfarin

Warfarin is generally considered the drug of choice. Nicoumalone and phenindione are seldom used. The baseline prothrombin time (PT) should be determined before the initial dose is given. The usual adult induction dose of warfarin is 10 mg daily for 2 days. The subsequent maintenance dose is considered on the basis of PT (reported as INR). The recommended therapeutic ranges are:

◆ INR 2–2.5 for DVT prophylaxis including surgery on high-risk patients;
◆ INR 2–3 for hip surgery, fractured femur operations, treatment of DVT or PE;
◆ INR 3–4.5 for recurrent DVT or PE.

INR is determined daily or on alternate days in early days of treatment, then at longer intervals (depending on response), then every 6–8 weeks. The daily maintenance dose of warfarin is 3–9 mg (taken at the same time each day).

Cautions

Caution should be taken in prescribing warfarin to patients with hepatic and renal disease and recent surgery. Drug interactions should be considered.

Complications

The most common complication is haemorrhage. When this occurs, the dose is omitted and the INR checked, and treatment is established on the basis of the INR. In the most severe cases treatment consists of vitamin K_1 and concentrate of factors II, IX, X and VII. When the INR is 4.5–7, treatment is discontinued and when the INR is >7 without haemorrhage, warfarin is discontinued and vitamin K_1 given. When unexpected bleeding occurs, even at therapeutic levels, unrecognized or subclinical disease (e.g. ulcerating bowel disease) is usually present.

Figure 15.1
Patient with nephrotic syndrome. Severe warfarin-induced skin necrosis.

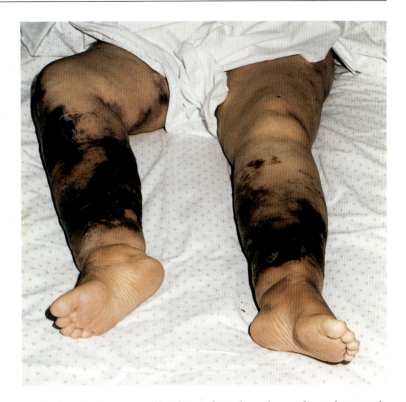

A devastating complication of oral anticoagulant therapy is haemorrhagic skin necrosis (**Figure 15.1**) which in the past was considered to be an allergic reaction. However, patients with this complication are deficient in protein C which may be the predisposing factor.

Warfarin is indicated mainly for secondary prophylaxis and treatment of DVT and PE.

Contraindications   Warfarin is contraindicated in pregnancy, peptic ulcer disease, severe hypertension and bacterial endocarditis.

Side effects   The main side effect is haemorrhage.

Nicoumalone (Sinthrome)   Nicoumalone has the same indications, cautions, contraindications and side effects as warfarin. This drug should also be avoided during breast feeding.

Dose   The dose given is 8–10 mg on the first day followed by 4–8 mg on the second day. The maintenance dose is usually 1–8 mg daily.

Phenindione (Dindevan)   Phenindione has the same indications, cautions, contraindications and side effects as warfarin. Side effects also include hypersensitivity reactions. This drug should also be avoided during breast feeding.

Dose   The dose given is 200 mg on the first day, followed by 100 mg on the second day. The maintenance dose is usually 50–150 mg daily.

ANTIPLATELET DRUGS   Antiplatelet drugs inhibit thrombus formation on the arterial side of the circulation where thrombi are formed by platelet aggregation and anticoagulants have little effect. Antiplatelet drugs have little effect in venous thromboembolism. So far only **aspirin** has been used extensively in practice but no significant results have been obtained by aspirin prophylaxis of DVT and PE. Therefore the role of aspirin in the prophylaxis of venous thromboembolism remains uncertain.

Indobufen   Indobufen prophylaxis (200 mg b.i.d. after 6 months of anticoagulation), in a prospective, 3-year study, has reduced the incidence of recurrent DVT after a major thrombotic episode of the lower limbs. However, the experience is limited.

FIBRINOLYTIC DRUGS   These drugs activate plasminogen to form plasmin which degrades fibrin, promoting the lysis of thrombi.

Cautions   There is a risk of bleeding from venepuncture or surgical wounds and risk of embolization from the clot.

Contraindications   Fibrinolytic drugs are contraindicated in patients with a history of recent haemorrhage, trauma, surgery, dental procedures, patients with coagulation defects, cerebrovascular disease, intestinal ulcerations, gynaecological problems causing bleeding, pulmonary disease with cavitation, acute pancreatitis, diabetic retinopathy, severe liver disease and oesophageal varices. In the case of streptokinase or anistreplase, previous allergic reactions to either drug or therapy with either drug from 5 to 12 months previously is a contraindication to use.

Side effects   Side effects of thrombolytic drugs are nausea, vomiting and back pain. Bleeding is usually limited at the site of injection but serious haemorrhage (i.e. cerebral) has been reported. With serious bleeding, treatment should be discontinued and administration of coagulation factors or antifibrinolytic drugs (aprotinin, tranexamic acid) may be required. Streptokinase and anistreplase may cause allergic reactions and anaphylaxis.

Alteplase (rt-Pa, tissue plasminogen activator) and anistreplase are indicated mainly for acute myocardial infarction and are not used for DVT and PE.

Streptokinase (Kabikinase, Streptase) is used in life-threatening DVT and PE. The treatment must be started very soon in order to be effective. Dose is by intravenous infusion, 250 000 units over 30 minutes, then 100 000 units every hour for up to 24–72 hours according to the clinical problem.

Urokinase (Ukidan, Urokinase) is used for thrombosed arteriovenous shunts and intravenous cannulas, thrombolysis in the eye, DVT and PE. It has the advantage of being non-immunogenic. Dose is by intravenous infusion, 4400 iu/kg over 10 minutes, then 4400 units/kg per hour for 12 hours in PE or for 12–24 hours in DVT. Bolus injection in PE may be given according to the data sheet.

Other drugs used in the prophylaxis of DVT and PE are dextran and Orgaran.

Dextran

Dextran 40 (Gentran 40, Rheomacrodex), administered by intravenous infusion has a molecular weight of about 40 000. Dextran 70 (Gentran 70, Macrodex) has a molecular weight of 70 000.

Indications

Dextran solutions are used in conditions associated with slow flow and for prophylaxis of post-surgical PE/DVT.

Cautions

Dextrans may interfere with blood group cross-matching or biochemical measurements. They should not be used to maintain plasma volume in situations such as burns or peritonitis where there is a loss of plasma proteins, water and electrolytes over a period of several days. In these situations plasma or plasma proteins should be given. It is necessary to correct dehydration before infusion and to give fluids during treatment. Severe congestive heart failure, renal failure, bleeding, thrombocytopenia and hypofibrinogenaemia may occur.

Dose

Dose is by intravenous infusion, initially 500–1000 ml, with the following doses according to the patient's condition.

Side effects

Rare anaphylactoid reactions have been observed.

Orgaran

Orgaran is a new antithrombotic, heparinoid drug (mixture of low molecular weight glycosaminoglycuronans including heparan sulphate, dermatan sulphate, and a small amount of chondroitin sulphate). This drug is chemically distinct from standard heparin and LMWHs. In hip surgery trials it has been used at the dosage of 750 anti-Xa units twice daily subcutaneously. The drug is considered as an effective antithrombotic agent in high-risk patients for the prevention of DVT with the potential advantage over unfractionated heparin and LMWH that it does not cross-react with antibodies to heparin or LMWH. The experience so far is limited as this compound is not widely available.

Other antithrombotic and heparinoid drugs

Other antithrombotic and heparinoid drugs are **defibrotide** and **mesoglycan**. However, information about their prophylactic action against DVT and PE is very limited.

DRUGS USED IN VENOUS INSUFFICIENCY

'Venoactive' drugs have been used for symptomatic relief in subjects with venous insufficiency. These drugs (**Table 15.2**) have very few important side effects and are safe. The claimed actions of these compounds are of three types:

◆ **symptomatic relief**;
◆ improvement of **venous tone**;
◆ decrease of the abnormally increased **capillary permeability and microcirculation alterations, leading to oedema formation**, observed in patients with venous insufficiency.

While subjective symptomatic relief has been observed in many patients with venous insufficiency, the claimed action on venous tone has not been clearly documented in humans. The action on the microcirculation and on the increased capillary filtration has been documented only in limited studies and it is possibly associated with the decrease in oedema formation and reduction in subjective symptoms. Large, double blind prospective studies are needed to

Table 15.2 Drugs used in venous insufficiency*

Name	Company
Arvenum 500	Stroder
Venoruton (Paroven)†	Zyma/Ciba-Geigy
Centellase	Corvi
Daflon 500	Servier
Doxium 500	OM
Essaven	Rhône-Polenc/Rorer
Flebosmil	Bouchara
Ginkor	Beaufour
Rutisan CE	Farmitalia
Troxerutin	Negma
Venobiase	Fournier

*Only the commercial name and producing company are included. This list is incomplete as several other drugs are available in different countries.

†Only one available in the UK.

confirm the role of chronic treatment or chronic prophylaxis with these drugs. Specifically, will these drugs,

- **used as treatments**, significantly improve signs and symptoms, particularly focusing on oedema development and control?
- **used as prophylaxis**, affect the evolution of chronic venous insufficiency?

The duration and cost-effectiveness of treatments may also be defined carefully (e.g. in comparison with elastic compression stockings). One important advantage of drug treatment is the possibility of using it in summer or when and where the average temperature is high, as an alternative to compression which is not well tolerated in such circumstances.

Oxpentifylline and defibrotide
Oxpentifylline (Trental) and defibrotide (Prociclide or Noravid) have been used to improve the healing of venous ulceration in limited prospective studies with good results. **Oral defibrotide** in subjects with chronic venous insufficiency improves the healing time of ulcerations, possibly as a consequence of the profibrinolytic action of the compound. **Oxpentifylline** possibly improves the healing of venous ulcers by its claimed action on the white cell accumulation in the venous ulcer area.

DRUGS USED FOR SCLEROTHERAPY
Ethanolamine oleate and sodium tetradecyl sulphate (STD, Trombovar) are used in sclerotherapy of varicose veins and **phenol** is used to treat haemorrhoids.

Cautions
Extravasation may cause necrosis of tissue.

Contraindications
Sclerotherapy should not be used in patients with recent DVT, superficial thrombophlebitis and patients unable to walk. Some authorities suggest avoiding sclerotherapy during treatment with oral contraceptives.

Dose
Ethanolamine oleate, 2–5 ml divided between three or four sites, is slowly injected in empty, isolated segments of varicose veins.

STD is injected, by the same procedure as for ethanolamine oleate, at a dose of 0.1–1.0 ml into each varicose segment. Up to 4–5 ml can be injected in the same session.

Lauromacrogols such as **laureth 9** (USAN)(**polidocanol, Aethoxysclerol**) are used at concentrations of 0.5%, 1%, 2% and 3% with the same procedures as described above. A very low concentration, according to the experience of the operator, is administered in small venous telangiectasias, an increasing concentration in small varicose veins, while higher concentrations (3%) are used only for large varicose veins and perforators.

Elastic compression (bandages and/or stockings) is an essential part of the treatment. *A simple rule easy to remember is that compression should be maintained for at least 1 week for veins of about 1 mm or less in diameter, for at least 2 weeks for veins of about 2 mm in diameter, and for at least 3 weeks for veins of 3 mm or more in diameter.*

Many other sclerosing agents are available (e.g. **Scleremo** (chrome alum) and other drugs) while some physicians use sclerosing solution directly made by themselves.

PHYSICAL TREATMENTS

Physical treatments of venous and lymphatic diseases are discussed in the relevant chapters. **Leg elevation, increased activity (e.g. walking), physiotherapy (e.g. manual lymph drainage),** and **weight loss** are all very effective measures to be regularly suggested to all patients with venous and lymphatic diseases.

Elastic compression is obtained with stockings or bandages. The two clinical applications of compression are **treatment** of signs and symptoms and acute (against DVT and PE) or chronic **prophylaxis** against the evolution of venous insufficiency. Compression when used as a treatment significantly improves signs and symptoms (particularly those associated with oedema). When used as a prophylactic method, compression inhibits the development of DVT and PE and may also inhibit the evolution of chronic venous insufficiency.

The most important disadvantage of **bandages** is that, to be effective, they have to be carefully placed by an expert (avoiding a tourniquet effect). Also, it is essential to replace them regularly (every 2 or 3 days), to ensure the appropriate compression, and most patients cannot do this by themselves.

Elastic stockings are very effective but again they should be tailored according to the patient with the problem that many elderly patients cannot put them on easily.

Graduated compression stockings are mainly used for DVT and PE prophylaxis. Other applications are the postoperative and post-sclerotherapy use as these stockings are more comfortable than bandages.

Pneumatic compression and sequential compression devices are mainly used for DVT and PE prophylaxis. However, chronic therapeutic applications include venous ulcerations and lymphoedema. Modified devices are often used for home treatment but the DVT and PE prophylaxis devices may also be successfully used.

LOCAL TREATMENT FOR VARICOSE VEINS AND ULCERATIONS

Most local treatments, available over the counter in many countries, have not been scientifically proven in prospective studies. The experience in this field is often different from country to country and it is difficult to give advice. While for varicose veins no logical local treatment is seriously advisable, a number of dressings, including hydrocolloid dressings, have been successfully used for venous ulcerations. The lack of scientific, prospective information does not exclude a possible positive action of many compounds. However, local treatment may produce severe reactions, complicating the clinical problem, and must therefore be used with care.

Note

Treatments, particularly drug treatments, have different means of application, dosages and brand names in different countries. Also, many drugs and products used in Europe are not used in the USA and UK and vice versa. The National Formulary (or the equivalent publication in each country) should always be consulted by the reader.

Further reading

Belcaro G *et al. Clinica Venosa.* Turin: Minerva Medica, 1993.
Belcaro G *et al. Vene.* Turin: Minerva Medica, 1993.
Belcaro G, Pierangeli A, Spartera C, Agus G. *Chirurgia Cardiaca e Vascolare.* Turin: Minerva Medica, 1994.
Belcaro G, Bollinger A, Hoffman U, Nicolaides AN. *Laser Doppler.* London: Med-Orion, 1994.
Bergan JJ, Yao JST (eds). *Surgery of the Veins.* Philadelphia: Grune & Stratton, 1984.
Bernstein EF. *Noninvasive Diagnostic Techniques in Vascular Disease.* St Louis, MI: Mosby, 1994.
Browse NL, Burnand KG, Thomas ML (eds). *Diseases of the Veins: Pathology, Diagnosis, and Treatment.* London: Arnold, 1988.
Comerota JT (ed). *Thrombolytic Therapy in Peripheral Vascular Disease.* New York: JB Lippincott, 1994.
Hirsch J, Genton E, Hull R. *Venous Thromboembolism.* Philadelphia: Grune & Stratton, 1981.
Enciclopedie Medico-Chirurgicale. Chirurgie Vasculaire Vol 2. Paris: Edition Techniques, 1993.
Pacific Vascular Symposium: Controversies in the Management of Venous Disorders. The Proceedings of the Straub Pacific Health Foundation, 1993.
Strandness DE Jr, Thiele BL. *Selected Topics in Venous Disorders: Pathophysiology, Diagnosis, and Treatment.* London: Futura, 1981.
Subcommittee on Reporting Standards in Venous Disease, Ad Hoc Committee on Reporting Standards, Society for Vascular Surgery, North America Chapter, International Society for Cardiovascular Surgery: Reporting standards in venous disease. *J Vasc Surg* 1988; 8: 172.
Tibbs DJ. *Varicose Veins and Related Disorders.* London: Butterworth-Heinemann, 1992.

Appendix

Forms that can be used by the clinician to define deep venous thrombosis or deep venous incompetence (1) and to mark superficial venous incompetence (2).

Form 1 DVT and/or deep venous incompetence

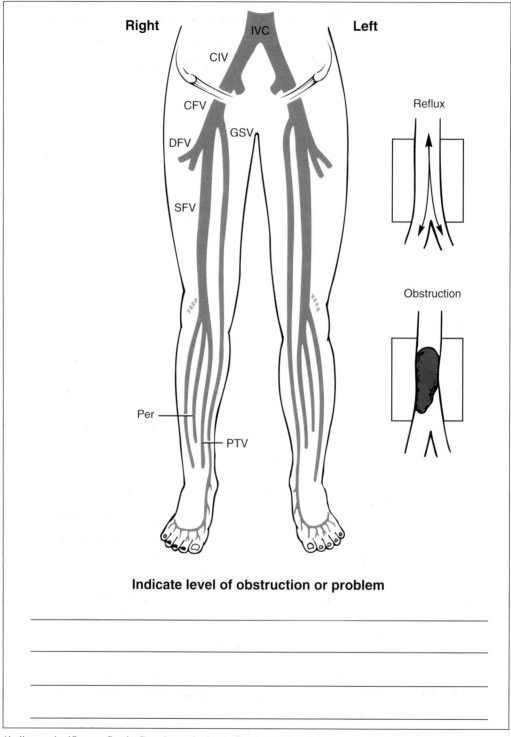

Right   IVC   **Left**

CIV

CFV

GSV

DFV

SFV

Per

PTV

Reflux

Obstruction

Indicate level of obstruction or problem

*indicates significant reflux by Doppler or duplex (reflux longer than 3 seconds on standing).
†indicates short lasting reflux (1–3 seconds).

Form 2 Superficial venous incompetence

Date _____ Mr/<u>Ms</u>_____

Referring Doctor or Unit _____

Right leg

Ant.   Post.

Section (cm)

— 11

— 10

— 9
— 8

— 7

— 6

— 5

— 4

— 3
— 2
— 1

Left leg

Ant.   Post.

Deep venous system

P	= **Patency**
O	= **Obstruction**
I	= **Incompetence**

☐ Cava

☐ Iliacs

☐ Common femoral

☐ Superficial femoral

☐ Popliteal

☐ Posterior tibial

☐ Distal veins

Duplex findings

_____

_____

_____

+ = **Reflux > 3 sec.**

x = **Reflux < 3 sec.**

Index

Page numbers in *italic* refer to figures and tables.